Pharmacy Calculations

3RD EDITION

$2\% = 2\text{ g}/100\text{ ml}$ $Tf = 9/5 * Tc + 32$ $2.5\text{ gm HC}/100\text{ gm}$

MARY F. POWERS
University of Toledo School of Pharmacy

JANET B. WAKELIN
Cuyahoga Community College

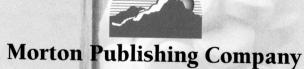

Morton Publishing Company
925 W. Kenyon Avenue, Unit 12
Englewood, Colorado 80110
www.morton-pub.com

BOOK TEAM

Publisher:	Douglas Morton
Editor/Production Coordinator:	Dona Mendoza
Assistant Editor:	Desiree Coscia
Copy Editor:	Elizabeth Budd
Cover & Design:	Bob Schram, Bookends
Composition:	Ash Street Typecrafters, Inc.

To the best of the Publisher's knowledge, the information presented in this book is correct and compatible with standards generally accepted for administering drugs. The reader is advised to consult the information material included with each drug or agent before administration. However, please note that you are reponsible for following your employer's and your state's policies, procedures, and guidelines.

The job description for pharmacy technicians varies by institution and state. Your employer and state can provide you with the most recent regulations, guidelines, and practices that apply to your work.

The Publisher of this book disclaims any responsibility whatsoever for any injuries, damages, or other conditions that result from your practice of the skills described in this book for any reason whatsoever.

Preface

The purpose of *Pharmacy Calculations* is to provide pharmacy technician students and pharmacy technicians with an educational tool to learn the types of calculations commonly encountered in community and institutional pharmacy. *Pharmacy Calculations* is a basic text that covers those topics encountered every day by pharmacy technicians. Although we initially developed the book as a text for pharmacy technician training programs, the book is also well-suited for use by pharmacy technicians working in the field.

The writing provides carefully worded explanations that are direct, easy to understand, and mathematically accurate. The material is presented in a straightforward manner to minimize confusion regarding what pharmacy calculations a technician should know. The format is logical and clear so that students can use the book for independent study or as part of a class. Graduates may use this book for the pharmacy technician certification exam.

This book allows students to develop a careful and systematic approach to pharmacy calculations. Because pharmacy calculations must be done with 100 percent accuracy, students are encouraged to use a calculator to solve the problems. Students are also invited to practice performing the calculations by hand so they can duplicate their work with 100 percent accuracy.

The third edition of *Pharmacy Calculations* has been revised and expanded on the basis of student and instructor feedback. It is in full color and includes new illustrations and pharmaceutical labels. Learning objectives have been included at the beginning of each chapter, along with a listing of key terms with their definitions. Additional examples of problems have been added to each chapter. A new chapter has been added: Chapter 37, "Dosage Calculations from Medication Labels." Also, additional problems have been added to some of the chapters. Finally, a set of 40 practice problems has been added at the end of the book to provide the student with additional practice on the concepts covered in the book.

Additionally, password-protected Instructors Ancillaries are available online. The ancillaries include:

- PowerPoint
- Lesson Plans
- Test Bank
- Answers to all the questions, along with helpful hints to solve the problems

Introduction

Pharmacy Calculations is divided into three main sections: basic arithmetic, calculations for community pharmacy, and calculations for institutional pharmacy.

- The chapters in Section 1, Basic Arithmetic, provide a foundation for the community pharmacy section and the institutional pharmacy section.

- The chapters in Section 2, Calculations for Community Pharmacy, include the types of calculations typically encountered in retail and outpatient settings.

- The chapters in Section 3, Calculations for Institutional Pharmacy, include the types of calculations typically encountered in hospital settings as well as other institutional settings.

The chapters are structured and written as follows:

- Each chapter begins with a set of learning objectives and key terms.

- The text in each chapter is direct, carefully worded, and concise.

- Each chapter includes real-world examples to show how to approach the problems.

- The problems at the end of each chapter are carefully worded and consistent with the material presented in each chapter.

- The number of examples and problems are adequate and appropriate to learn the calculations.

- The way the material is presented allows the student to isolate any chapter in the community pharmacy or institutional pharmacy sections and focus on a specific topic of interest.

- Students are encouraged to use a calculator for routine calculations so that they can focus on comprehending and understanding the concepts that are presented.

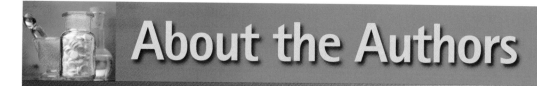

About the Authors

Mary F. Powers, Ph.D., R.Ph., is Associate Professor of Pharmacy Practice at the University of Toledo College of Pharmacy in Toledo, Ohio. She received her pharmacy degree from the University of Toledo College of Pharmacy and her Doctor of Philosophy in Medical Sciences degree from the Medical College of Ohio, Toledo, Ohio. Powers has extensive experience in community pharmacy practice and has also served as the Pharmacy Technician Program Coordinator at Mercy College of Northwest Ohio, Toledo, Ohio, as an adjunct faculty member at the Medical College of Ohio, and has been involved in teaching pharmacy technicians since 1998.

Janet B. Wakelin, MRPharmS, is the retired Director of the Pharmacy Technician Training Program at Cuyahoga Community College in Cleveland, Ohio. She received her pharmacy degree from Aston University, Birmingham, England. Wakelin has community and hospital experience as a Registered Pharmacist in England and as a Certified Technician in the United States. She served as Treasurer for the Pharmacy Technician Educators Council (PTEC) from 1994 to 1998, and has been involved in teaching pharmacy technicians since 1991. She now lives with her husband in Charlotte, North Carolina.

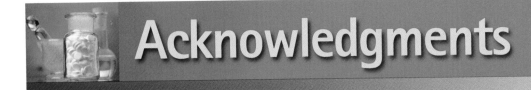

Acknowledgments

We want to take this opportunity to thank Doug Morton, whose sponsorship makes this book possible. We also give special thanks to Dona Mendoza, Project Manager at Morton Publishing, for all of her help and support in each edition of the book. Thanks also to Desiree Coscia at Morton Publishing for her work to obtain permissions, labels, and illustrations for the third edition of the book.

We are grateful to Douglas Scribner, Chairman of the Pharmacy Technician Program at Central New Mexico Community College, for his suggestions on the initial effort and review of the first edition for errors. Thank you also to Karen Snipe, Marsha Sanders, and Kim Ballow for their helpful suggestions on the initial effort. Thank you to Dr. Gerhard Lind, Retired Chairman, Department of Chemistry, Metropolitan State College of Denver, for his review of the problems that were new to the second edition for errors. Thank you to Dr. David Bright, Assistant Professor of Pharmacy Practice, Ohio Northern University, for his review of the problems that were new to the third edition for errors.

Finally, thank you to supporting colleagues, family, and friends, including: David Wakelin, Ph.D., for checking the institutional math; Nigel Wakelin, Pharm.D., for the chemotherapy examples; Sarah Martin for reading institutional sections with the eyes of a non-pharmacy person; Mary's dog Cimmy, who has provided immeasurable support for each edition of the book; and Judith Jones, Ph.D., because without her support, this book would not be possible.

Sincerely,
Mary F. Powers and Janet B. Wakelin

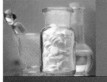

Contents

Basic Arithmetic

2% = 2 g/100 ml   Tf = 9/5*Tc+32   2.5 gm HC/100 gm

In This Section

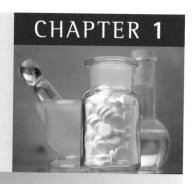

Numeral Systems Used in Pharmacy

CHAPTER 1

LEARNING OBJECTIVES

After completing this chapter, the student will be able to:

1 Explain the meaning of Roman numerals and Arabic numerals

2 Convert Roman numerals to Arabic numerals

3 Convert Arabic numerals to Roman numerals

4 Determine the number of tablets or capsules needed to fill a prescription that has the quantity written in Roman numerals

KEY TERMS

Roman numerals: numeral system based in ancient Rome that uses letters and combinations of letters

Arabic numerals: numeral system in common use today based on the ten digits 0, 1, 2, 3, 4, 5, 6, 7, 8, 9

ARITHMETIC IS THE BRANCH OF MATHEMATICS in which numbers are used to solve problems. There are many systems in the world for writing numbers. The system for writing numbers that is widely used throughout the world today is based on the number 10 and is known as the Arabic system. In the Arabic system, the position a symbol occupies helps determine the value of the symbol. For example, in 333, the 3 on the right means three, but the 3 in the middle means three tens and the 3 on the left means three hundreds.

Rx CAPSULE Arabic numerals are the ten digits commonly used in math problems.

Another system for writing numbers that is sometimes used in pharmacy is the Roman numeral system. Roman numerals are expressed by letters of the alphabet and are rarely used today except for formality or variety.

The principles for reading Roman numerals are:

■ A letter repeated once or twice repeats its value that many times (XXX = 30, CC = 200, etc.).

■ One or more letters that is placed after another letter of greater value increases the greater value by the amount of the smaller (VI = 6, LXX = 70, MCC = 1200, etc.).

■ A letter placed before another letter of greater value decreases the greater value by the amount of the smaller (IV = 4, XC = 90, CM = 900, etc.).

The following common Roman numerals correspond to the following values in the Arabic system:

Letter	Value	Letter	Value	Letter	Value	Letter	Value
I	1	VII	7	XL	40	C	100
II	2	VIII	8	L	50	D	500
III	3	IX	9	LX	60	M	1000
IV	4	X	10	LXX	70		
V	5	XX	20	LXXX	80		
VI	6	XXX	30	XC	90		

Reading Roman numerals requires a different approach than reading Arabic numerals, and generally the position of the Roman numeral is not as important as it is in the Arabic system.

EXAMPLE

Convert the Roman numeral XXIX to the Arabic numeral.

XX = 20

IX = 9

XXIX = 20 + 9 = 29

EXAMPLE

Convert the Arabic numeral 67 to the Roman numeral.

LX = 60

VII = 7

Combining the two Roman numerals yields LXVII

EXAMPLE

Convert the Roman numeral XIV to the Arabic numeral.

X = 10

IV = 4

XIV = 10 + 4 = 14

EXAMPLE

Convert the Arabic numeral 122 to the Roman numeral.

C = 100

XX = 20

II = 2

Combining the Roman numerals yields CXXII

EXAMPLE

How many tablets are needed for the following prescription?

William M. Fox, MD
1234 Main St
Anytown, Ohio 12345
(321) 123-4567

Name _____ Jone Doe _____ Date _____ 5/11/2010 _____

Address _____

Tylenol #3   XXX

Sig: ꝷ-ii q 4-6 h prn pain

William Fox MD
AF1234567

NR

For this prescription, the quantity is expressed in Roman numerals and XXX = 30.
Therefore, 30 tablets are needed to fill the prescription.

Rx CAPSULE   Some prescribers use Roman numerals for the number of tablets or capsules to dispense.

PRACTICE PROBLEMS

STUDENT NAME _____

DATE _____ COURSE NUMBER _____

Convert the following Roman numerals to Arabic numerals:

1. XIX   = 19
    10 9

2. XC   = 90
    10 100
      100 - 10

3. CCC   = 300

4. XXXII   = 32

5. XLIV   = 64
    10 50   5
    60 + 5 = 1

6. XXII   = 22

7. VII   = 7

8. IV   = 4
    5 - 1

9. III   = 3

10. XIX   = 19
    10 10
    10 + 10 - 1

11. XXXIII = 33

12. CIX   = 109
    100 10
    100 + 10 - 1

13. II   = 2

14. VIII   = 8

15. XXIV   = 24
    10 10 5
    20 + 5 - 1

16. XXXIV   = 34
    30 + 5 - 1

17. XLIII   = 63
    50
    10

18. XXVIII = 28
    20

19. XIII   = 13

20. XXIX   = 29
    20 + 10 - 1

Convert the following Arabic numerals to Roman numerals:

21. 10   =   X   31. 4   =   IV

22. 20   =   X X   32. 7   =   VII

23. 30   =   X X X   33. 12   =   XII

                                    (50 - 10)

24. 40   =   ~~XXXX~~ XL   34. 16   =   XVI

25. 50   =   L   35. 22   =   XXII

26. 15   =   XV   36. 36   =   XXXVI

27. 100   =   C   37. 49   =   IL

28. 200   =   CC   38. 57   =   LVII

29. 300   =   CCC   39. 150   =   CL

                                                        1000 - 100

30. 1000   =   M   40. 900   =   CM

Numerators, Denominators, and Reciprocals of Fractions

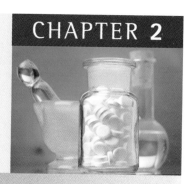

CHAPTER 2

LEARNING OBJECTIVES

After completing this chapter, the student will be able to:

1 Define the terms *fraction, numerator,* and *denominator*

2 Explain the relationship between the numerator and the denominator in a fraction

3 Define the term *reciprocal*

4 Explain why a denominator cannot be zero

5 Convert fractions to decimals

6 Convert decimals to fractions

KEY TERMS

Whole numbers: expressions in the Arabic system for the numbers 1, 2, 3, 4, 5, and so on

Fraction: expression in the Arabic system to represent part of a whole

Numerator: the top number in a fraction

Denominator: the bottom number in a fraction

Decimal: a special type of fraction in which the denominator is a number that is a power of 10

Equivalent fractions: fractions that represent the same amount

Reciprocals: two fractions that when multiplied together equal 1

IN THE ARABIC SYSTEM, fractions are used to indicate amounts that fall in between whole numbers. In other words, a fraction represents part of a whole. The division of two whole numbers can also be represented by a fraction. The two parts of a fraction are the numerator and denominator. The denominator (the number below the bar) tells us how many parts the whole is divided into, and the numerator (the number above the bar) tells us how many of those parts exist.

> **℞ CAPSULE**   Remember, the numerator is the top number of a fraction and the denominator is the bottom number (you can think: the Denominator is Down).

In a fraction, the numerator can be zero, but the denominator cannot be zero. Division by zero is undefined, therefore, no denominator can be zero.

One way to think of a fraction is as division that hasn't been completed yet.

EXAMPLE

3/4

You can read this fraction as three-fourths, three over four, or three divided by four.

A decimal is a special type of fraction in which the denominator is a number that is a power of 10. In other words, for decimals, the denominators could be 10, 100, or 1000, etc.)

The following decimals correspond to the following fractions in the Arabic system

Decimal	Fraction
0.1	1/10
0.01	1/100
0.001	1/1000
0.0001	1/10,000
0.00001	1/100,000
0.000001	1/1,000,000

℞ CAPSULE   Never use terminal zeros following the decimal point for doses expressed in whole numbers. 1 mg could be misread as 10 mg if a terminal zero was added following the decimal point.

℞ CAPSULE   Always use zero before a decimal when the dose is less than a whole unit. Without the preceding zero, 0.5 mg could be misread as 5 mg.

Understanding decimals is important in pharmacy. Often doses of medications are expressed in terms of decimals.

EXAMPLE

Express the milligram (mg) strength of each drug below in the form of a fraction:

Synthroid 0.025 mg = 25/1000 mg
Synthroid 0.050 mg = 50/1000 mg
Synthroid 0.075 mg = 75/1000 mg
Synthroid 0.088 mg = 88/1000 mg
Synthroid 0.10 mg = 1/10 mg
Synthroid 0.1112 mg = 1112/10,000 mg
Synthroid 0.125 mg = 125/1000 mg
Synthroid 0.137 mg = 137/1000 mg
Synthroid 0.150 mg = 150/1000 mg
Synthroid 0.175 mg = 175/1000 mg
Synthroid 0.20 mg = 2/10 mg
Synthroid 0.30 mg = 3/10 mg
Lanoxin 0.25 mg = 25/100 mg

Fractions can be converted to decimals by performing the division using a calculator:

3/4 = 0.75

EXAMPLE

Here are some other fractions and their decimal equivalents. Remember, you can find the decimal equivalent of any fraction by dividing the numerator by the denominator.

2/5 = 0.4
3/5 = 0.6
4/5 = 0.8

There are many ways to write fractions. Fractions that represent the same number are called equivalent fractions. For example, 1/2, 2/4, and 4/8 are all equal. To determine if two fractions are equal, use a calculator and divide. If the answer is the same, then the fractions are equal.

Reciprocals of Fractions

Reciprocals are two different fractions that when multiplied together equals 1. Every fraction has a reciprocal (except those fractions with zero in the numerator). The easiest way to find the reciprocal of a fraction is to switch the numerator and denominator, or just flip the fraction over.

To find the reciprocal of a whole number, just put 1 over the whole number.

℞ CAPSULE   To see if two fractions are reciprocals, simply multiply them by each other. If the result is 1, then the fractions are reciprocals.

EXAMPLES

The reciprocal of 2 is 1/2

The reciprocal of 3 is 1/3

The reciprocal of 4 is 1/4

The reciprocal of 2/3 is 3/2

PRACTICE PROBLEMS

STUDENT NAME _____

DATE _____ COURSE NUMBER _____

Use a calculator to convert the following fractions to decimals:

1. 1/2   =   0.5

2. 1/4   =   0.25

3. 2/4   =   0.5

4. 2/5   =   0.4

5. 1/10   =   0.1

6. 1/8   =   0.125

7. 1/12   =   0.083 = Repeated

8. 1/20   =   0.05

9. 1/100   =   0.01

10. 1/1000 =   0.001

11. 3/8   =   0.375

12. 3/4   =   0.75

13. 4/5   =   0.8

14. 1/3   =   0.33

15. 7/12   =   0.583

16. 1/7   =   (0.143) 0.14285714286

17. 5/11   =   0.4545 (0.45)

18. 5/6   =   0.83

19. 2/9   =   0.22

20. 5/18   =   0.27 (0.28)

21. 3/7   =   (0.43) 0.4285714285

22. 3/11   =   0.2727 (0.273)

23. 3/21   =   (0.143) 0.14285714286

24. 3/33   =   0.0909 (0.091)

25. 5/35   =   0.1428571486 (0.143)

26. 7/43   =   0.16279069767 (0.163)

27. 9/55   =   0.16363 (0.164)

28. 13/63   =   0.20634920635 (0.2063)

29. 15/71   =   0.21126760563 (0.2113)

30. 23/83   =   0.27710843373 (0.28)

Determine the reciprocal of the following fractions:

31. 1/2   = $\dfrac{2}{1} = 2$

32. 1/4   = $\dfrac{4}{1} = 4$

33. 2/4   = $\dfrac{4}{2} = 2$

34. 2/5   = $\dfrac{5}{2} = 2\frac{1}{2}$

35. 1/10   = $\dfrac{10}{1} = 10$

36. 1/8   = $\dfrac{8}{1} = 8$

37. 1/12   = $\dfrac{12}{1} = 12$

38. 1/20   = $\dfrac{20}{1} = 20$

39. 1/100   = $\dfrac{100}{1} = 100$

40. 1/1000   = $\dfrac{1000}{1} = 1000$

41. 3/8   = $\dfrac{8}{3} = 2\frac{2}{3}$

42. 3/4   = $\dfrac{4}{3} = 1\frac{1}{3}$

43. 4/5   = $\dfrac{5}{4} = 1\frac{1}{4}$

44. 1/3   = $\dfrac{3}{1} = 3$

45. 7/12   = $\dfrac{12}{7} = 1\frac{5}{7}$

46. 1/7   = $\dfrac{7}{1} = 7$

47. 5/11   = $\dfrac{11}{5} = 2\frac{1}{5}$

48. 5/6   = $\dfrac{6}{5} = 1\frac{1}{5}$

49. 2/9   = $\dfrac{9}{2} = 4\frac{1}{2}$

50. 5/18   = $\dfrac{18}{5} = 3\frac{3}{5}$

51. 3/13   = $\dfrac{13}{3} = 4\frac{1}{3}$

52. 3/23   = $\dfrac{23}{3} = 7\frac{2}{3}$

53. 5/7   = $\dfrac{7}{5} = 1\frac{2}{5}$

54. 5/12   = $\dfrac{12}{5} = 2\frac{2}{5}$

55. 5/37   = $\dfrac{37}{5} = 7\frac{7}{5}$

56. 7/48   = $\dfrac{48}{7} = 6\frac{6}{7}$

57. 7/51   = $\dfrac{51}{7} = 7\frac{2}{7}$

58. 9/23   = $\dfrac{23}{9} = 2\frac{5}{9}$

59. 11/52   = $\dfrac{52}{11} = 4\frac{8}{11}$

60. 23/83   = $\dfrac{83}{23} = 3\frac{14}{23}$

CHAPTER 3

Reducing Fractions to Lowest Terms

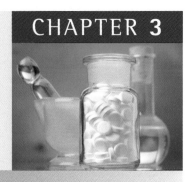

LEARNING OBJECTIVES

After completing this chapter, the student will be able to:

1 Explain how to reduce a fraction to lowest terms

2 Define the terms *prime factor* and *common factor*

3 Determine the greatest common factor of a fraction

4 Reduce fractions to lowest terms

KEY TERMS

Simplifying a fraction: reducing a fraction so the numerator and denominator are the smallest whole numbers possible

Greatest common factor: the whole number that both numerator and denominator can be divided by to reduce the fraction

Prime factor: a whole number divisible by only 1 and itself

Canceling: dividing the numerator a denominator of a fraction by all common factors

TO REDUCE A FRACTION TO LOWEST TERMS, also known as simplifying a fraction, divide the numerator and denominator by their greatest common factor. The greatest common factor is a whole number and both the numerator and denominator can be divided by this number (factor). Some fractions are already in lowest terms if there is no factor common to the numerator and denominator.

> ℞ CAPSULE   Reducing a fraction is also known as simplifying the fraction.

The steps to reduce a fraction to its lowest terms are:

1. Identify the prime factors (a prime factor is a whole number that is divisible by only 1 and itself) of the numerator and denominator.

2. Find the factors common to both the numerator and denominator.

3. Divide the numerator and denominator by all common factors (this is called canceling).

EXAMPLE

Reduce the fraction to lowest terms.

  15/35

1. List the prime factors of the numerator and denominator.

    Numerator: 1,3,5

    Denominator: 1,5,7

2. Divide by, or cancel, the factor of 5 that is common to both the numerator and denominator.

3. You're left with a 3 in the numerator and a 7 in the denominator.

    Numerator: 15/5 = 3

    Denominator: 35/5 = 7

Therefore 15/35 reduced to lowest terms is 3/7.

R̶ CAPSULE   Reducing a fraction will not change its value.

EXAMPLE

Reduce the fraction 9/36 to lowest terms.

1. List the prime factors in the numerator and denominator.

    Numerator: 1, 3

    Denominator: 1, 2, 3

    *Note that 3 × 3 = 9, and 9 is also a factor of 36.

2. Divide by or cancel the factor of 9 that is common to both the numerator and denominator.

    Numerator: 9/1 = 1

    Denominator: 36/9 = 4

3. You're left with 1 in the numerator and 4 in the denominator. Therefore, 9/36 reduced to lowest terms is 1/4.

EXAMPLE

Reduce the fraction 30/110 to lowest terms.

1. List the prime factors in the numerator and denominator.

    Numerator: 1, 2, 3, 5

    Denominator: 1, 2, 5, 11

    *Note that both 2 and 5 are common factors of 30 and 110, so you can multiply 2 × 5 = 10.

2. Divide both the numerator and denominator by 10.

3. You're left with 3 in the numerator and 11 in the denominator. Therefore, 30/110 reduced to lowest terms is 3/11.

PRACTICE PROBLEMS

STUDENT NAME _____

DATE _____ COURSE NUMBER _____

Reduce the following fractions to lowest terms:

1. 3/9 $\frac{3 \div 3}{9 \div 3}$ = _____ 1/3 _____

2. 6/24 $\frac{6 \div 6}{24 \div 6}$= _____ 1/4 _____

3. 2/4 $\frac{2 \div 2}{4 \div 2}$= _____ 1/2 _____

4. 2/16 $\frac{2 \div 2}{16 \div 2}$= _____ 1/8 _____

5. 6/10 $\frac{6 \div 2}{10 \div 2}$ $\frac{3}{5}$= _____ 3/5 _____

6. 12/36 $\frac{12 \div 6}{36 \div 6} = \frac{2}{6}$ _____ 2/6 _____

7. 18/54 $\frac{18 \div 6}{54 \div 6}$= _____ 3/9 $\div 3$ 1/3 _____

8. 10/220 $\frac{10 \div 10}{220 \div 10}$= _____ 1/22 _____

9. 25/125 $\div 25$ = _____ 1/5 _____

10. 65/75 $\div 5$ = _____ 13/15 _____

11. 21/35 $\div 7$ = _____ 3/5 _____

12. 72/90 $\div 9$ = _____ 8/10 $\div 2$ 4/5 _____

13. 36/27 $\div 9$ = _____ 4/3 = 1 1/3 _____

14. 15/75 $\div 15$ = _____ 1/5 _____

15. 16/24   = _____ 2/3 _____

16. 9/12 $\div 3$ = _____ 3/4 _____

17. 6/20 $\div 2$ = _____ 3/10 _____

18. 16/40 $\div 4$ = _____ 4/10 $\div 2$ 2/5 _____

19. 24/30 $\div 6$ = _____ 4/5 _____

20. 14/36 $\div 2$ = _____ 7/18 _____

21. 5/11   = _____ 5/11 _____

22. 0/25   = _____ 0 _____

23. 75/100 $\div 25$ = _____ 3/4 _____

24. 22/55 $\div 11$ = _____ 2/5 _____

25. 60/75 $\div 5$ = _____ 12/15 _____

26. 30/36 $\div 6$ = _____ 5/6 _____

27. 7/28 $\div 7$ = _____ 1/4 _____

28. 26/39 $\div 13$ = _____ 2/13 _____

29. 27/56   = _____ 27/56 _____

30. 34/51 $\div 17$ = _____ 2/3 _____

31. 36/48   =   _____

32. 24/100   =   _____

33. 16/32   =   _____

34. 30/45   =   _____

35. 28/42   =   _____

36. 12/35   =   _____

37. 66/84   =   _____

38. 14/63   =   _____

39. 30/70   =   _____

40. 6/51   =   _____

41. 125/500   =   _____

42. 25/100   =   _____

43. 25/150   =   _____

44. 50/500   =   _____

45. 270/2700   =   _____

46. 65/585   =   _____

47. 73/292   =   _____

48. 82/164   =   _____

49. 79/237   =   _____

50. 17/102   =   _____

51. 19/285   =   _____

52. 18/81   =   _____

53. 24/36   =   _____

54. 112/280   =   _____

55. 59/118   =   _____

56. 77/154   =   _____

57. 121/605   =   _____

58. 63/135   =   _____

59. 42/72   =   _____

60. 33/77   =   _____

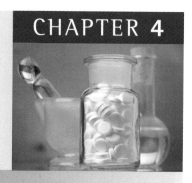

Adding and Subtracting Fractions

CHAPTER 4

LEARNING OBJECTIVES

After completing this chapter, the student will be able to:

1 Define the term *least common denominator*

2 Find equivalent fractions with common denominators for a pair of fractions that do not have common denominators

3 Solve problems that require addition of fractions

4 Solve problems that require subtractions of fractions

KEY TERMS

Common denominator: two fractions have the same denominator

Least common denominator: the common denominator for two fractions is the smallest possible whole number

IN ORDER TO ADD OR SUBTRACT FRACTIONS, the fractions must have the same denominator (called common denominators). To add or subtract fractions that have common denominators, you simply add or subtract the numerators and write the sum or difference over the common denominator.

In order to add or subtract fractions with different denominators, you must first find equivalent fractions with common denominators:

1. Find the smallest multiple for the denominator of both numbers.

2. Rewrite the fractions as equivalent fractions with the smallest multiple of both numbers as the denominator.

When working with fractions, the smallest multiple of both denominator numbers is called the least common denominator.

EXAMPLE

   1/2 + 1/3

The smallest multiple for the denominator of both numbers is 6.

   1/2 = (1 × 3)/(2 × 3) = 3/6

   1/3 = (1 × 2)/(3 × 2) = 2/6

The problem can now be rewritten as follows:

3/6 + 2/6

Because the denominators are equal, you only need to add the numerators to get the answer.

(3 + 2)/6 = 5/6

EXAMPLE

4/5 − 1/3

The smallest multiple for the denominator of both numbers is 15.

4/5 = (4 × 3)/(5 × 3) = 12/15

1/3 = (1 × 5)/(3 × 5) = 5/15

The problem can now be rewritten as follows:

12/15 − 5/15

Because the denominators are equal, you only need to subtract the numerators to get the answer.

(12 − 5)/15 = 7/15

℞ CAPSULE   Remember, before you can add or subtract fractions, you must first create common denominators.

EXAMPLE

3/11 + 4/22

The smallest multiple for the denominator of both numbers is 22.

3/11 = (3 × 2) / (11 × 2) = 6/22

4/22 = 4/22

The problem can be rewritten as follows:

6/22 + 4/22

Add the numerators to get the answer.

(6 + 4)/22 = 10/22

Reduce to lowest terms by dividing the numerator and denominator by 2.

5/11

EXAMPLE

1/4 + 1/3 + 1/5

The smallest multiple for the denominator of all three numbers is 60.

1/4 = (1 × 15) / (4 × 15) = 15/60

1/3 = (1 × 20) / (3 × 20) = 20/60

1/5 = (1 × 12) / (5 × 12) = 12/60

The problem can be rewritten as follows:

15/60 + 20/60 + 12/60

Add the numerators to get the answer.

47/60

PRACTICE PROBLEMS

STUDENT NAME _____

DATE _____ COURSE NUMBER _____

Calculate the following fractions:

1. 1/3   +   1/3   = __2/3__

2. 1/8   +   3/8   = __4/8__ = 2/4 = 1/2

3. 2/3   −   1/3   = __1/3__

4. 5/8   −   3/8   = __2/8__ = 1/4

5. 1/5   +   3/5   = __4/5__

6. 7/8   −   3/8   = __4/8__ = 1/2

7. 1/3   −   1/5   = __2/15__

    ×5   ×3

    5/15 − 3/15

8. 4/25   +   1/5   = ____ 9/25 ____

4/25 + 5/25   (×5)

9. 1/8   +   3/16   = _____

10. 7/8   −   1/4   = _____

11. 3/8   +   3/5   = _____

12. 1/5   +   3/5   = _____

13. 2/7   +   3/7 + 1/7 = _____

14. 4/15   +   6/15   = _____

15. 1/8   +   2/8 + 7/8   = _____

16. 1/2   +   3/5   = _____

17. 3/8   +   11/12   =   _____

18. 5/21   +   5/28   =   _____

19. 2/3   +   1/6   +   5/12   =   _____

20. 5   +   7/10   +   3/1000   =   _____

21. 6/10   −   4/10   =   _____

22. 5/6   −   4/6   =   _____

23. 3/25   +   12/25   =   _____

24. 3/14   −   2/14   =   _____

25. 7/5   −   3/5   =   _____

26. 1/20   +   3/20   =   _____

27. 11/15   –   7/15   =   _____

28. 5/8   +   4/27   +   1/48   =   _____

29. 6   +   1/100   +   3/10   =   _____

30. 1/10   +   3/10   +   9/1000   =   _____

31. 3/5   +   1/5   +   3/10   +   7/10   =   _____

32. 3/4   +   1/4   +   1/8   +   5/8   =   _____

33. 1/12   +   5/12   +   1/3   +   2/3   =   _____

34. 1/9   +   4/9   +   1/3   +   1/18   =   _____

35. 1/2   +   4/5   +   1/10   +   1/20   =   _____

36. 2/9   +   4/9   +   1/2   +   5/18   =   _____

37. 1/7   +   4/7   +   6/35   +   1/35   =   _____

38. 12/19   +   14/38   +   1/19   +   1/38   =   _____

39. 11/12   +   1/3   +   2/3   +   1/24   =   _____

40. 1/5   +   4/5   +   1/10   +   1/20   =   _____

41. 1/2   +   3/4   +   1/3   +   1/12   =   _____

42. 1/3   +   1/4   +   1/12   +   1/24   =   _____

43. 1/2   +   1/3   +   1/4   +   1/24   =   _____

44. 11/99 +   4/9 +   11/33 +   1/18   =   _____

45. 10/90 +   4/9 +   1/3   +   1/18   =   _____

46. 1/8   +   1/4 +   1/2   +   3/8   =   _____

47. 1/3   +   1/6 +   1/9   +   1/18   =   _____

48. 1/2   +   1/9 +   1/36   +   1/18   =   _____

49. 1/5   +   3/10 +   3/20   +   3/40   =   _____

50. 1/19   +   1/38 +   1/76   +   1/152   =   _____

Multiplying and Dividing Fractions

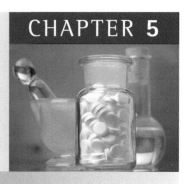

CHAPTER 5

LEARNING OBJECTIVES

After completing this chapter, the student will be able to:

1 Describe the procedure for multiplying fractions

2 Solve problems that require multiplying fractions

3 Describe the procedure for dividing fractions

4 Solve problems that require dividing fractions

KEY TERMS

Multiplying fractions: mathematical operation to obtain the products of the numbers in the numerators and products of the numbers in the denominators

Dividing fractions: mathematical operation to find the reciprocal of the fraction you are dividing by and then multiplying the fractions

UNLIKE ADDING AND SUBTRACTING, when multiplying fractions you do not need a common denominator. To multiply fractions:

1. Multiply the numerators of the fractions to get the new numerator.

2. Multiply the denominators of the fractions to get the new denominator.

3. Simplify the result if possible.

EXAMPLE

Determine $1/3 \times 2/5$.

1. Multiply the numerators $(1 \times 2) = 2$.

2. Multiply the denominators $(3 \times 5) = 15$.

3. The resulting fraction is 2/15 (already simplified).

Dividing by fractions is just like multiplying fractions, but there is one additional step to convert the fraction you are dividing by, to its reciprocal. To divide fractions:

1. Find the reciprocal of the fraction you are dividing by.

2. Multiply the first fraction times the reciprocal determined in step 1.

3. Simplify the resulting fraction by reducing to lowest terms, if possible.

Important: Because division by zero is undefined, the number 0 has no reciprocal.

Sometimes, it is necessary to solve for a fractional amount of another fraction. For example, what is 1/2 of 1/4? You can think of this problem visually.

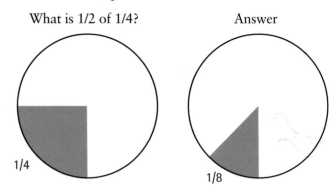

Mathematically, you can simply determine 1/2 of 1/4 by multiplying both fractions

1. Multiply both numerators $(1 \times 1) = 1$.

2. Multiply both denominators $(2 \times 4) = 8$.

3. The resulting fraction is 1/8.

EXAMPLE

Divide 24 by 1/4

1. Find the reciprocal of the fraction you are dividing by. The reciprocal of 1/4 is 4/1.

2. Multiply $24/1 \times 4/1 = 96$.

3. Because 96 is a whole number, the answer is already simplified.

EXAMPLE

Divide 1/3 by 1/5

1. Find the reciprocal of the fraction you are dividing by. The reciprocal of 1/5 is 5/1.

2. Multiply $1/3 \times 5/1 = 5/3$.

3. Simplify 5/3 to 1 2/3.

Divide 3 by 1/2.

1. First find the reciprocal of the fraction you are dividing by (the reciprocal of 1/2 is 2/1)

2. Then multiply $3 \times 2/1 = 6$.

3. The answer is 6.

Rx CAPSULE   Remember, you can only divide by non-zero fractions.

PRACTICE PROBLEMS

STUDENT NAME _____

DATE _____ COURSE NUMBER _____

Multiply the following fractions:

1. 1/3   of   1/3   =   _1/9_

2. 1/8   of   3/8   =   _3/64_

3. 2/3   of   1/3   =   _2/9_

4. 5/8   of   3/8   =   _15/64_

5. 1/5   of   3/5   =   _3/25_

6. 7/8   of   3/8   =   _21/64_

7. 0/4   of   5/6   =   _5/6_

8. 1/5   of   3/4   =   _3/20_

9. 5/6   of   5/6   =   _25/36_

10. 2/3   of   4/7   =   _8/21_

11. 3/4   of   3/4   =   _____

12. 1/9   of   2/3   =   _____

13. 1/3   ×   1/5   =   _____

14. 4/25   ×   1/5   =   _____

15. 1/8   ×   3/16   =   _____

16. 7/8   ×   1/4   =   _____

17. 3/8   ×   3/5   =   _____

18. 7/16   ×   1/4   =   _____

19. 1/9   ×   4/9   =   _____

20. 2/1   ×   5/1   =   _____

21. 7/10   ×   1/5   =   _____

22. 4/13   ×   2/5   ×   6/7   =   _____

23. $9/100 \quad \times \quad 1 \quad \times \quad 3 \quad = $ _____

24. $3/11 \quad \times \quad 0/8 \quad \times \quad 6/7 \quad = $ _____

25. $1/3 \quad \times \quad 1/20 \quad \times \quad 1/8 \quad = $ _____

26. $1/3 \quad \times \quad 1/4 \quad \times \quad 1/5 \quad \times \quad 3/7 \quad = $ _____

27. $4/7 \quad \times \quad 3/5 \quad \times \quad 1/9 \quad \times \quad 1/4 \quad = $ _____

28. $1/8 \quad \times \quad 3/8 \quad \times \quad 1/2 \quad \times \quad 1/3 \quad = $ _____

29. $3/7 \quad \times \quad 1/2 \quad \times \quad 1/4 \quad \times \quad 1/3 \quad = $ _____

30. $5/8 \quad \times \quad 1/3 \quad \times \quad 2/3 \quad \times \quad 3/7 \quad = $ _____

31. $3/7 \quad \times \quad 2/7 \quad \times \quad 1/2 \quad \times \quad 1/3 \quad = $ _____

32. $1/5 \quad \times \quad 1/3 \quad \times \quad 1/4 \quad \times \quad 1/8 \quad = $ _____

33. $3/8 \quad \times \quad 2/3 \quad \times \quad 1/3 \quad \times \quad 3 \quad = $ _____

34. $5/8 \quad \times \quad 1/3 \quad \times \quad 1/2 \quad \times \quad 3/8 \quad = $ _____

35. $1/9 \quad \times \quad 1/2 \quad \times \quad 1/3 \quad \times \quad 3/7 \quad = $ _____

Divide the following fractions:

36. 1/3   divided by   1/3   =   _____

37. 1/8   divided by   3/8   =   _____

38. 2/3   divided by   1/3   =   _____

39. 5/8   divided by   3/8   =   _____

40. 1/5   divided by   3/5   =   _____

41. 7/8   divided by   3/8   =   _____

42. 1/3   divided by   1/5   =   _____

43. 4/25   divided by   1/5   =   _____

44. 1/8   divided by   3/16   =   _____

45. 7/8   divided by   1/4   =   _____

46. 3/8   divided by   3/5   =   _____

47. 3/4   divided by   8/5   =   _____

48. 2/3   divided by   1/2   =   _____

49. 16/27   divided by   8/9   =   _____

50. 5/15   divided by   5   =   _____ $\frac{5}{15}$ $\frac{1}{5}$ $\frac{5}{75}$

51. 9/10   divided by   9/10   =   _____

52. 7/5   divided by   5/7   =   _____

53. 3/5   divided by   0   =   _____

54. 0   divided by   7/8   =   _____

55. 5/24   divided by   3/8   =   _____

56. 7/48   divided by   14/16   =   _____

57. 14/20   divided by   7/4   =   _____

58. 25   divided by   1/5   =   _____

59. 30   divided by   1/10   =   _____

60. 50   divided by 1/2   = _____

61. 4   divided by 1/2   = _____

62. 5   divided by 1/5   = _____

63. 7   divided by 1/14   = _____

64. 12   divided by 3/8   = _____

65. 14   divided by 2/7   = _____

66. 20   divided by 1/10   = _____

67. 35   divided by 3/10   = _____

68. 100   divided by 1/3   = _____

69. 300   divided by 3/8   = _____

70. 1000 divided by 1/5   = _____

Writing Fractions in Decimal Form

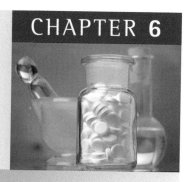

LEARNING OBJECTIVES

After completing this chapter, the student will be able to:

1 Explain how decimal fractions are written

2 Express in words the value of decimal fractions

3 Express in numbers the value for decimal fractions that are given in words

4 Convert fractions to decimals

KEY TERMS

Decimal number system: a number system that uses a notation so each number is expressed in base 10 by using one of the first nine integers or 0 in each place and letting each place value be a power of 10

Power: the number of times that a number occurs as a factor in a product as indicated by an exponent

IN THE DECIMAL NUMBER SYSTEM, the value of a digit depends on its place or location in the number. Each place has a value of 10 times the place to its right. Numbers to the left of the decimal point are separated into groups of three digits using commas. As you move right from the decimal point, each place value is divided by 10.

Zero and the counting numbers (1, 2, 3, etc.) make up the set of whole numbers. But not every number is a whole number. The decimal system allows us to write numbers that are fractions as well as whole numbers by using a symbol called the decimal point.

You read the decimal number 105.599 as "one hundred five and five hundred ninety-nine thousandths." The "th" at the end of a word means a fraction part (or a part to the right of the decimal point). You can also read this number as "one hundred five point five nine nine."

EXAMPLE

Eight hundred = 800

Eight hundredths = 0.08

EXAMPLE

Write the number three hundred twenty-three and four tenths in decimal form.

323.4

EXAMPLE

Write the number five hundred fifty-five thousandths in decimal form.

0.555

EXAMPLE

Write 13 506/1000 in decimal form.

13.506

EXAMPLE

Write the number three hundred fifty and forty-four hundredths in decimal form.

350.44

EXAMPLE

Write the number four point two six in decimal form.

4.26

EXAMPLE

Write the number fifty six thousandths in decimal form.

0.056

EXAMPLE

Express the number 5.02 in words.

Five and two hundredths

or

Five point zero two

EXAMPLE

Express 1,400.02 in words.

One thousand four hundred and two hundredths

or

One thousand four hundred point zero two

℞ CAPSULE   Tenfold medication errors are defined as errors in which the dose was 10 times greater or smaller than the correct dose. Tenfold or decimal point medication errors are especially dangerous for patients! Use extreme caution when working with decimals.

PRACTICE PROBLEMS

STUDENT NAME _____

DATE _____   COURSE NUMBER _____

Write the following as decimal numbers:

1. Thirty-two hundredths   =   _____

2. Thirty-three thousandths   =   _____

3. Two hundred thirty-seven thousandths   =   _____

4. Thirty-five and one hundred fifty-three thousandths   =   _____

5. Five hundred three and thirty-two hundredths   =   _____

6. Eighty-six hundredths   =   _____

7. Ninety-nine thousandths   =   _____

8. Three tenths   =   _____

9. Fourteen thousandths   =   _____

10. Seventeen hundredths   =   _____

11. Six and twenty-eight hundredths   =   _____

12. Sixty and twenty-eight thousandths   =   _____

13. Seventy-two and three hundred ninety-two thousandths   =   _____

14. Eight hundred fifty and thirty-six ten-thousandths   =   _____

Write the following decimal numbers in words:

15. 0.5   =   _____

16. 0.93   =   _____

17. 5.06   =   _____

18. 32.58   =   _____

19. 71.06   =   _____

20. 35.078   =   _____

21. 7.003   =   _____

22. 18.102   =   _____

23. 50.008   =   _____

24. 607.607 =   _____

Write the following decimals as fractions (do not reduce to lowest terms):

25. 593.86   =   _____   36. 1.35   =   _____

26. 0.63   =   _____   37. 3.3   =   _____

27. 0.75   =   _____   38. 4.53   =   _____

28. 0.88   =   _____   39. 6.08   =   _____

29. 0.73   =   _____   40. 10.353   =   _____

30. 0.2   =   _____   41. 20.354   =   _____

31. 0.35   =   _____   42. 31.451   =   _____

32. 0.47   =   _____   43. 49.326   =   _____

33. 0.66   =   _____   44. 51.118   =   _____

34. 0.41   =   _____   45. 101.101   =   _____

35. 0.03   =   _____

Rounding Decimals and Significant Figures

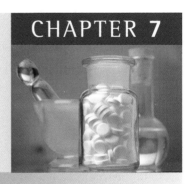

LEARNING OBJECTIVES

After completing this chapter, the student will be able to:

1 Describe the procedure for rounding decimals

2 Demonstrate rounding decimals to the nearest tenth and hundredth

3 Define significant figures

4 Explain the importance of using significant figures in pharmacy calculations

5 List the four rules for assigning significant figures

KEY TERMS

Rounding decimals: a process to eliminate unnecessary decimal numbers

Significant figures: when performing calculations that include measured quantities, the number of digits in a calculated number corresponding to the sensitivity of the measuring device

---

SOMETIMES, AFTER MULTIPLYING DECIMAL FRACTIONS or after converting a fraction to a decimal fraction, the number of decimal places is too large to be manageable. Extra numbers can be confusing and can also contribute to errors in calculations. Therefore, it is often useful and advisable to round off decimals.

To round off decimals:

■ Find the digit for place value you want (the "rounding digit") and look at the digit just to the right of it.

■ If that digit is less than 5, do not change the rounding digit, and drop all digits to the right.

■ If that digit is greater than or equal to five, add one to the rounding digit and drop all digits to the right.

EXAMPLE

To round the number 15,732.7343 to the nearest thousandth:

1. Find the rounding digit. This is 4.

2. Look one digit to the right, at the digit in the ten-thousandths place which is "3".

3. See that 3 is less than 5, so leave the number "4," then drop the digits to the right of 4.

This gives 15,732.734.

EXAMPLE

To round 622.1352 to the nearest hundredth:

1. Find the rounding digit, "3."

2. Look at the digit one place to right, "5." 5 = 5.

3. Because the rule states if the number to the right of the rounding digit is greater than or equal to 5, add one to the rounding digit, and drop all digits to the right of it.

Therefore, this number needs to be rounded up. Add one to the rounding digit and remove all the rest of the digits to the right of it. The result is 622.14

EXAMPLE

To round the number 47.5464 to the nearest tenth:

1. Find the rounding digit. This is 5.

2. Look one digit to the right at the digit in the hundredths place which is 4.

3. See that 4 is less than 5, so leave the number "5", then drop the digits to the right of 5.

Answer: 47.5

EXAMPLE

To round the number 49.504 to the nearest whole number:

1. Find the rounding digit. This is 9.

2. Look one place to the right and find the number 5.

3. Because the rule states if the number to the right of the rounding digit is greater than or equal to 5, add one to the rounding digit and drop all digits to the right of it.

Answer: 50

Significant Figures

A significant digit is one that is actually measured. The number of significant digits in a measurement depends on the measuring device used and the sensitivity of that measuring device. When a calculation involves measurements with different numbers of significant figures in the entries or terms that are added, subtracted, multiplied, etc., the answer should have the same number of significant digits as the entry or term with the least number of significant figures in the measurement.

Rules for assigning significant figures:

■ Digits other than zero are always significant.

■ Final zeros after a decimal point are always significant.

■ Zeros between two other significant digits are always significant.

■ Zeros used only to space the decimal are never significant.

EXAMPLE

Determine the number of significant figures in 3.4502 grams.

Because zeros between two other significant digits are always significant, the number of significant figures is 5.

EXAMPLE

Determine the number of significant figures in 3.40 grams.

Because final zeros after a decimal point are always significant, the number of significant figures is 3.

EXAMPLE

Determine the number of significant figures in 0.036 grams.

Because zeros used only to space the decimal are never significant, the number of significant figures is 2.

EXAMPLE

Determine the number of significant figures in 2.5 ml (if the volume was measured using a device that measures accurately to the nearest tenth of a milliliter).

Because digits other than zero are always significant, the number of significant figures is 2.

EXAMPLE

Determine the number of significant figures in 20.0 ml (if the volume was measured using a device that measures accurately to the nearest tenth of a milliliter).

Because the final zero after a decimal point is always significant, the number of significant figures is 3.

R̥ CAPSULE When performing pharmaceutical calculations, the importance of showing all significant figures is generally outweighed by the occasional disastrous consequences of including them. For example, showing trailing zeros after a decimal point can contribute to misreading the dose that results in a tenfold dosing error.

PRACTICE PROBLEMS

STUDENT NAME _____

DATE _____ COURSE NUMBER _____

Round the following decimal numbers to the nearest hundredth:

1. 132.35789   = _____   6. 2.339   = _____

2. 6.993928394   = _____   7. 1.006   = _____

3. 2.357895733   = _____   8. 3.232323232   = _____

4. 235,121.34764   = _____   9. 101.234   = _____

5. 132,424,324.351   = _____   10. 136.567   = _____

Round off each decimal number to the nearest tenth:

11. 80.015   = _____   16. 0.037   = _____

12. 7.555   = _____   17. 3.2323   = _____

13. 180.009   = _____   18. 44.444   = _____

14. 37.6666   = _____   19. 365.365   = _____

15. 14.3332   = _____   20. 0.245   = _____

Round off each decimal number to the nearest whole number:

21. 32.134   = _____   27. 2.95   = _____

22. 55.556   = _____   28. 3.25   = _____

23. 109.421   = _____   29. 145.2   = _____

24. 0.76   = _____   30. 3.33   = _____

25. 100   = _____   31. 4.12   = _____

26. 1.00   = _____   32. 54.329   = _____

33.   100.01   =   _____   37.   512.8   =   _____

34.   325.2   =   _____   38.   1000.9   =   _____

35.   467.1   =   _____   39.   2001.09   =   _____

36.   479.9   =   _____   40.   345.59   =   _____

Determine the number of significant figures in each measurement:

41. 6.222 g   =   _____

42. 0.123 kg   =   _____

43. 12.0 ml   =   _____

44. 0.030 g   =   _____

45. 20.05 grams   =   _____

CHAPTER 8

Adding and Subtracting Decimal Numbers

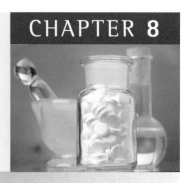

LEARNING OBJECTIVES

After completing this chapter, the student will be able to:

1 Perform addition of decimal numbers

2 Perform subtraction of decimal numbers

KEY TERMS

Adding decimals: mathematical operation similar to adding whole numbers, except terms must be lined up so that all decimal points are in a vertical line

Subtracting decimals: mathematical operation similar to subtracting whole numbers, except terms must be lined up so that all the decimal points are in a vertical line

ADDING AND SUBTRACTING DECIMALS is just like adding and subtracting whole numbers. When adding and subtracting decimals, it is very important to line up the terms so that all the decimal points are in a vertical line.

To add decimal numbers:

1. Put the numbers in a vertical column so the decimal points are aligned.

2. Add each column of digits, starting on the right and work left. If the sum of a column is more than 10, "carry" the digits to the next column on the left.

3. Place the decimal point in the answer directly below the decimal points in the numbers.

EXAMPLE

Step 1

$$
\begin{array}{r}
324.5678 \\
+\ \ \ 1.2345 \\
\hline
3 \text{ (carry the 1)}
\end{array}
$$

Step 2

$$
\begin{array}{r}
324.5678 \\
+\ \ \ 1.2345 \\
\hline
23 \text{ (carry the 1)}
\end{array}
$$

Step 3

```
   324.5678
+    1.2345
─────────────
          023 (carry the 1)
```

Step 4

```
   324.5678
+    1.2345
─────────────
        .8023
```

Step 5

```
   324.5678
+    1.2345
─────────────
       5.8023
```

Step 6

```
   324.5678
+    1.2345
─────────────
      25.8023
```

Step 7

```
   324.5678
+    1.2345
─────────────
     325.8023
```

EXAMPLE

Step 1

```
  40.25
+ 1.035
────────
      5
```

Step 2

```
  40.25
+ 1.035
────────
     85
```

Step 3

```
  40.25
+ 1.035
────────
    .285
```

Step 4

```
  40.25
+ 1.035
────────
   1.285
```

Step 5

```
  40.25
+ 1.035
────────
  41.285
```

To subtract decimal numbers:

1. Put the numbers in a vertical column so the decimal points are aligned.

2. Subtract each column, starting on the right and working left. If the digit being subtracted in a column is larger than the digit above it, "borrow" a digit from the next column to the left.

3. Place the decimal point in the answer directly below the decimal points in the terms.

EXAMPLE

Step 1

$$
\begin{array}{r}
32.255 \\
-\ 1.203 \\
\hline
2
\end{array}
$$

Step 2

$$
\begin{array}{r}
32.255 \\
-\ 1.203 \\
\hline
52
\end{array}
$$

Step 3

$$
\begin{array}{r}
32.255 \\
-\ 1.203 \\
\hline
.052
\end{array}
$$

Step 4

$$
\begin{array}{r}
32.255 \\
-\ 1.203 \\
\hline
1.052
\end{array}
$$

Step 5

$$
\begin{array}{r}
32.255 \\
-\ 1.203 \\
\hline
31.052
\end{array}
$$

EXAMPLE

$24.0 - 0.75$

℞ CAPSULE   To set this up, it is helpful to add an additional zero following 24.0 to hold the place.

Step 1

$$
\begin{array}{r}
24.00 \\
-0.75 \\
\hline
5
\end{array}
$$

Step 2

$$
\begin{array}{r}
24.00 \\
-0.75 \\
\hline
.25
\end{array}
$$

Step 3

$$
\begin{array}{r}
24.00 \\
-0.75 \\
\hline
3.25
\end{array}
$$

Step 4

$$
\begin{array}{r}
24.00 \\
-0.75 \\
\hline
23.25
\end{array}
$$

PRACTICE PROBLEMS

STUDENT NAME _____

DATE _____ COURSE NUMBER _____

Add the following decimal fractions:

1. $0.6 + 0.4 + 1.3$ = _____

2. $5 + 6.1 + 0.4$ = _____

3. $0.59 + 6.91 + 0.05$ = _____

4. $3.488 + 16.593 + 25.002$ = _____

5. $37.02 + 25 + 6.4 + 3.89$ = _____

6. $4.0086 + 0.034 + 0.6 + 0.05 \quad = \quad$ _____

7. $43.766 + 9.33 + 17 + 206 \quad = \quad$ _____

8. $52.3 + 6 + 21.01 + 4.005 \quad = \quad$ _____

9. $2.0051 + 0.2006 + 5.4 + 37 \quad = \quad$ _____

10. $5 + 2.37 + 463 + 10.88 \quad = \quad$ _____

11. $2 + 3 + 3.5 + 4.6 + 5.5 \quad = \quad$ _____

12. 2.4 + 1.3 + 1.5 + 4.3 + 15.9   = _____

13. 1.1 + 2.2 + 3.3 + 4.4 + 5.5   = _____

14. 12 + 3.5 + 3.3 + 144 + 155   = _____

15. 20 + 30 + 4.55555 + 400.6 + 501.5   = _____

16. 2.2 + 3.3 + 5.5 + 6.6 + 7.5 + 7.7   = _____

17. 122 + 301 + 55.5 + 6.5 + 701.5 + 7.007   = _____

18. 2 + 3 + 5 + 6.6663 + 7.501 + 12.0007   = _____

19. 12.2 + 23.3 + 55.5 + 36.6 + 7.0005 + 7.7   = _____

20. 212 + 3.0003 + 5.005 + 6.06 + 7.12 + 12.8   = _____

21. 354.2312	22. 224.0021	23. 5223.2312
+ 5.1092	+ 6.4444	+ 65.3217

24. 22375.23	25. 34.2312875
+ 5.92	+ 22.1092

Subtract the following decimal fractons:

26. 5.2 − 3.76   =   _____

27. 17.83 − 8.9   =   _____

28. 29.5 − 13.61   =   _____

29. 1.0057 − 0.03   =   _____

30. 78.015 − 13.068   =   _____

31. 22.418 − 17.524   =   _____

32. 4.8 − 0.0026   =   _____

33. 31.009 − 0.534   =   _____

34. 4 − 1.0566   =   _____

35. 40.718 − 6.532   =   _____

36. 3.8 − 2.12   =   _____

37. 5 − 0.002   =   _____

38. 13.01 − 12   =   _____

39. 123 − 0.001   =   _____

40. 117.2 − 117   =   _____

41. 145.45 − 0.44   =   _____

42. 136.3 − 125.2   =   _____

43. 111 − 0.01   =   _____

44. 110 − 0.1   =   _____

45. 345.34 − 1.32   =   _____

46.   354.2312   47.   224.0012   48.   5223.2312
      −   5.1092   −   6.4444   −   65.3217
      _____   _____   _____

49.   22375.23   50.   34.2312875
      −   5.92   − 22.1092
      _____   _____

CHAPTER 9

Multiplying and Dividing Decimal Numbers

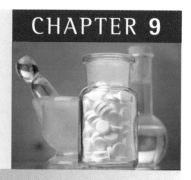

LEARNING OBJECTIVES

After completing this chapter, the student will be able to:

1 Define the terms *product, dividend, divisor,* and *quotient*

2 Perform multiplication with decimal numbers

3 Perform division with decimal numbers

KEY TERMS

Product: the number that results when numbers are multiplied together

Dividend: in division, the number that is divided

Divisor: in division, the number that the dividend is divided by

Quotient: the number that results when one number is divided by another

MULTIPLICATION IS OFTEN INDICATED by an " × " inserted between numbers. Another way to indicate multiplication is to separate adjacent numbers by parentheses. Multiplication can also be indicated by a "·" or "*" that is inserted between numbers.

To multiply decimal numbers:

1. Multiply the numbers as if they were whole numbers.

2. Line up the numbers on the right in the same way you would if there were no decimal points.

3. Start at the right side and multiply each digit in the top number by each digit in the bottom number.

4. Add the product resulting from multiplying each digit of the bottom number.

5. Place the decimal point in the answer so that the number of decimal places in the answer equals the total number of decimal places in both numbers that were multiplied together.

EXAMPLE

47.2×5.5:

$$
\begin{array}{r}
47.2 \text{ (has 1 decimal place)} \\
\times \quad 5.5 \text{ (has 1 decimal place)} \\
\hline
2360 \\
+\ 2360 \\
\hline
259.60 \text{ (2 decimal places)}
\end{array}
$$

> **℞ CAPSULE** When multiplying decimal numbers, you can start by multiplying normally and ignoring the decimal points. To determine the decimal point in the answer, count the decimal places in the numbers that are multiplied and the answer will have as many decimal places as the two original numbers combined.

EXAMPLE

Find the product of 9.683×6.1.

$$
\begin{array}{r}
9.683 \text{ (has 3 decimal places)} \\
\times \quad 6.1 \text{ (has 1 decimal place)} \\
\hline
9683 \\
+\ 58098 \\
\hline
59.0663 \text{ (3 + 1 = 4 decimal places)}
\end{array}
$$

Sometimes it is necessary to perform division with decimal numbers. In division, one number called the dividend is divided by another number called the divisor to result in the quotient.

If the divisor is a whole number and the divided is a decimal, you can divide the numbers as if they were whole numbers except you must mark the decimal place in the decimal.

$$
\text{divisor} \overline{)\text{dividend}}^{\text{quotient}}
$$

When the dividend is a decimal and the divisor is a whole number:

1. Mark the place of the decimal in the dividend before you start dividing.

2. Divide each step as you would for whole numbers.

3. Repeat until the steps of division are complete.

4. Check your answer by multiplying the quotient by the divisor. The answer should be the dividend.

EXAMPLE

Divide 3.64 by 4.

Step 1

$$4\overline{)3.64}$$

Step 2

$$
\begin{array}{r}
0.9 \\
4\overline{)3.64} \\
36 \\
\hline
4
\end{array}
$$

Step 3

$$
\begin{array}{r}
0.91 \\
4\overline{)3.64} \\
36 \\
\hline
4 \\
4 \\
\hline
0
\end{array}
$$

You can check your answer to see whether the product of the quotient and divisor equals the dividend:

$0.91 \times 4 = 3.64$

> **℞ CAPSULE** When dividing decimals, first use long division without the decimal point. Then, when determining your answer, simply reinsert the decimal point in the answer and put the decimal point in the answer directly above the decimal point in the dividend.

PRACTICE PROBLEMS

STUDENT NAME _____

DATE _____ COURSE NUMBER _____

Use a calculator to convert the following fractions to decimals:

1. $(0.6)(0.7)$ = _____

2. $(0.3)(0.8)$ = _____

3. $(0.2)(0.2)$ = _____

4. $(0.3)(0.3)$ = _____

5. $8(2.7)$ = _____

6. $4(9.6)$ = _____

7. 1.4(0.3)   = _____

8. 1.5(0.6)   = _____

9. (0.2)(0.02)   = _____

10. (0.3)(0.03)   = _____

11. 5.4(0.02)   = _____

12. 7.3(0.01)   = _____

13. 0.23(0.12)   = _____

14. (0.15)(0.15) = _____

15. (8.1)(0.006) = _____

16. 7.1(0.008) = _____

17. 0.06(0.01) = _____

18. 0.25(0.01) = _____

19. (3.23)(2.32) = _____

20. 14.5(15.4) = _____

21. 122.1(212.12)   = _____

22. 3.3 * 4.4   = _____

23. 5.52 * 4.1   = _____

24. 3.741 * 2.122   = _____

25. 15.41 * 12.12   = _____

26. 144.44 * 2.3   = _____

27. 513.312 * 0.5   = _____

28. 25.12 * 0.2   = _____

29. 12.2 * 0.3   = _____

30. 36.63 * 1.5   = _____

31. 122 * 4.2   = _____

32. 42.24 * 42.24   = _____

33. 135.1 * 10   = _____

34. 146.63 * 100   = _____

35. 1.235 * 1000   = _____

36. 4.222 * 0.01   = _____

37. 31.31 * 13.1   = _____

38. 10 * 0.1   = _____

39. 100 * 0.01   = _____

40.   35.23
       × 22.12
     _____

41.   253.424
       ×   4.2
     _____

42.   2.5
         × 3.27
       _____

43.   527.225
      ×   2.1
   _____

44.   2.38795
      ×   1.1
   _____

45.   326.311
      × 2.113
   _____

46.   1.21
      × 3.333
   _____

47. 2.44 ÷ 4   = _____

48. 32.12 ÷ 2   = _____

49. 183.12 ÷ 3   = _____

50. 466.2 ÷ 3   = _____

51. 666.6 ÷ 6   = _____

52. 30.25 ÷ 5.5   = _____

53. 9.36 ÷ 3.6   = _____

54. 11.25 ÷ 1.5   = _____

55. 40.3225 ÷ 6.35   = _____

56. 315.5 ÷ 63.1   = _____

57. 38.19 ÷ 5.7   = _____

58. 365.75 ÷ 5.5   = _____

59. 8.1 ÷ 9   = _____

60. 24.2 ÷ 4.4   = _____

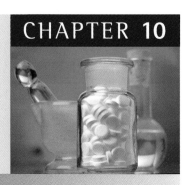

CHAPTER 10

Using Ratios and Proportions or Dimensional Analysis to Solve Pharmacy Calculations

LEARNING OBJECTIVES

After completing this chapter, the student will be able to:

1 Define the terms *ratio, proportion,* and *dimensional analysis*

2 Explain how to solve problems using ratio and proportion

3 Explain how to solve problems using dimensional analysis

4 Demonstrate how to solve common pharmacy problems using ratio and proportion and dimensional analysis

KEY TERMS

Ratio: expression to compare two numbers

Proportion: expression for two ratios that are equal

Dimensional analysis: method based on ratios and proportions to solve mathematical problems

MOST CALCULATIONS IN PHARMACY can be solved using either of two techniques: ratio and proportion or dimensional analysis.

Ratio and Proportion

Ratios are used to make comparisons between two things. When you express ratios in words, you use the word "to." For example, you say "the ratio of something to something else."

A ratio can be written in several different ways: as a fraction, using the word "to," or with a colon.

EXAMPLE

The following expressions all represent the ratio "3 to 5":

3/5

3 to 5

3:5

Equal ratios are two different ratios that may include different numbers when expressed as fractions, but can be reduced to the same fraction. To find an equal ratio, multiply or divide each term in the ratio by the same number (but not zero).

EXAMPLE

Express the ratio 1:4 as a fraction.

1/4

EXAMPLE

If you divide both terms in the ratio 3:6 by the number three, then you get the equal ratio, 1:2. Examples of other equal ratios include:

3:6 = 12:24 = 6:12 = 15:30

These can also be expressed as:

3/6 = 12/24 = 6/12 = 15/30

EXAMPLE

Identify two equal ratios for 100:10.

100:10 = 50:5 = 10:1 (There are others.)

Proportions

A proportion is a name given to a statement that two ratios are equal. Proportions can be written in two ways:

■ As two equal fractions, a/b = c/d

■ Using a colon, a:b = c:d

When two ratios are equal, then the products of the means (or middle numbers) equals the products of the extremes (or outside numbers).

℞ CAPSULE   When solving problems using ratios and proportions, remember the product of the means is equal to the product of the extremes.

EXAMPLE

For the proportion a:b = c:d, b × c (means) = a × d (extremes).

The proportion 20/30 = 2/3 is read as "twenty is to thirty as two is to three."

In problems involving proportions, you can test the products of the means and extremes to test whether two ratios are equal and form a proportion.

The ratios 20/30 and 2/3 form a proportion because the product of the means equals the product of the extremes.

30 × 2 = 60

20 × 3 = 60

℞ CAPSULE   When solving problems using ratios and proportions, be sure to carefully label the units of the numbers. Mistakes are sometimes made when numbers with different units are confused.

EXAMPLE

Solve for y:

4:y = 8:32

Because the product of the means equals the product of the extremes,

8y = 4 × 32
8y = 128
 y = 128/8 = 16

EXAMPLE

Solve for y:

3:27 = 2:y
   54 = 3y
    y = 18

EXAMPLE

Solve for y:

3:36 = y:12
  36y = 36
    y = 1

Dimensional Analysis

Dimensional analysis is a useful method scientists employ to check the validity of scientific equations and calculations. For some very complicated problems in science, sometimes, dimensional analysis is the only way to find the right answer! Dimensional analysis can also be used for most pharmacy calculations either to check your work, or, once you've mastered the technique, may be the best way to get the correct answer to your problem. Some people find dimensional analysis to be extremely helpful for complicated pharmaceutical calculations.

In science, the dimension of an object tells you what sort of quantity it is. In science, there are four basic dimensions: length, mass, time, and electrical charge. Similarly, in pharmacy we can think of pharmaceutical quantities in terms of the "dimensions" such as weight, volume, dose, dosage form, and time (day[s]).

To solve a problem using dimensional analysis, you need to first identify what information is provided by the problem as well any conversion factors that you will need to solve the problem. Terms that are equal to each other are written in the form of a fraction. For example, if 250 mg = 1 dose, you would write this as a fraction:

$$\frac{250 \text{ mg}}{1 \text{ dose}} \quad \text{or} \quad \frac{1 \text{ dose}}{250 \text{ mg}}$$

Because both fractions are equal to 1, you can write either term in the numerator. Once you have written all of the information, you need to solve the problem in the form of fractions. To do this, you simply set up a series of fractions (making sure to label each term!) in an equation so that when the fractions are multiplied, all units will cancel out, except the units you need for your answer.

EXAMPLE

You can use dimensional analysis to determine how many capsules are needed to fill a prescription for amoxicillin 250 mg/capsule, one capsule three times per day for seven days:

Use dimensional analysis to solve this problem:

$$\frac{capsule}{250 \ mg} \times \frac{250 \ mg}{dose} \times \frac{3 \ doses}{day} \times 7 \ days = 21 \ capsules$$

1. Start by setting up a dimensional analysis equation so the units you want in the final answer (the capsule) is in the numerator of the first fraction of the dimensional analysis equation.

2. Set up the next fraction in the dimensional analysis equation so the units of the numerator of the second fraction are the same as the units of the denominator of the first fraction (that is, so the units cancel when the fractions are multiplied).

3. Set up the next fraction in the dimensional analysis equation so the units of the numerator of the third fraction are the same as the units of the denominator of the second fraction (again, so the units cancel when the fractions are multiplied).

4. Set up the next fraction in the dimensional analysis equation so the units of the numerator of the fourth fraction are the same as the units of the denominator of the third fraction (again, so the units cancel when the fractions are multiplied).

5. Multiply the fractions!

Important: Always remember to check your work!

For this example, when all fractions are multiplied together, all units cancel except the capsule units (which is in the numerator). When using dimensional analysis, you need to be careful to make sure that the numerator (not the denominator) contains the units you need to solve the problem.

EXAMPLE

A prescription is written for amoxicillin 300 mg per dose. Use dimensional analysis to determine how many milliliters of amoxicillin suspension 250 mg/5 ml would deliver the required dose.

Because you are solving for milliliters, start by placing a term with ml in the numerator.

$$\frac{5 \ ml}{250 \ mg} \ \bigg| \ \frac{300 \ mg}{} \ = \ 6 \ ml$$

EXAMPLE

How many doses are in a bottle of 150 ml of amoxicillin 250 mg/5 ml if each dose is 5 ml?

$$\frac{Dose}{5 \ ml} \ \bigg| \ \frac{150 \ ml}{bottle} \ = \ 30 \ doses$$

> ℞ CAPSULE   Placing the units you want in the final answer in the numerator of the first term of the dimensional analysis set up helps to ensure your answer will be in the correct units. Also, units can be canceled only when identical units appear in both the numerator and denominator.

PRACTICE PROBLEMS

STUDENT NAME _____

DATE _____ COURSE NUMBER _____

Use ratio and proportion or dimensional analysis to solve the following problems:

1. In the proportion 5/8 = 25/40:

    a. The extremes are _____ and _____.

    b. The means are _____ and _____.

Fill in the blank for each pair of ratios to form a proportion:

2. 2/3   and   4/_____

3. 5/7   and   15/_____

4. 3/6   and   1/_____

5. 5/10   and   7/_____

6. 2/8   and   3/_____

7. _____/3   and   4/6

8. _____/8   and   3/24

9. _____/12   and   5/6

10. _____/4   and   6/8

11. _____/5   and   10/25

12. _____/6   and   10/12

13. _____/7   and   6/42

14. _____/15   and   2/5

15. _____/5   and   4/10

16. 3/5   and   _____/100

17. 125/1000   and   _____/8

18. 3/8   and   375/_____

19. 2/3   and   _____/12

20. How many tablets will be taken in seven days if a prescription order reads zafirlukast 20 mg/tablet, one tablet twice a day?

        _____

21. How many capsules will be taken in three days if a prescription order reads tetracycline 250 mg/capsule, one capsule four times a day?

        _____

22. How many tablets will be taken in five days if a prescription order reads sucralfate 1 g/tablet, one tablet four times a day?

        _____

23. How many tablets will be taken in 10 days if a prescription order reads zaleplon 5 mg/tablet, one tablet daily at bedtime?

        _____

24. How many tablets will be taken in 30 days if a prescription order reads methylphenidate 10 mg/tablet, one tablet three times a day?

        _____

25. How many capsules are needed to fill a prescription for 30 days for zidovudine 100 mg/capsules, three capsules twice daily?

        _____

26. How many tablets are needed to fill a prescription for 34 days for nabumetone 500 mg/tablet, one tablet twice daily?

        _____

27. How many tablets will be taken in 10 days if a prescription order reads metoclopramide 5 mg/tablet, one tablet three times a day?   _____

28. How many tablets will be taken in 10 days if a prescription order reads rabeprazole 20 mg/tablet, one tablet twice a day?   _____

29. How many tablets will be taken in seven days if a prescription order reads albuterol 2 mg/tablet, one tablet four times a day?   _____

30. How many tablets will be taken in two days if a prescription order reads promethazine 12.5 mg/tablet, one tablet three times a day?   _____

31. How many tablets will be taken in five days if a prescription order reads fluphenazine 1 mg/tablet, one tablet three times a day?   _____

32. How many capsules are needed to fill a prescription for 14 days for ampicillin 500 mg/capsule, one capsule four times a day?   _____

33. How many tablets are needed to fill a prescription for 30 days for primadone 250 mg/tablet, one tablet three times a day?   _____

34. How many tablets are needed to fill a prescription for 34 days for acarbose 50 mg/tablet, one tablet three times a day?

        _____

35. How many capsules are needed to fill a prescription for 34 days for prazosin 1 mg/capsules, two capsules three times a day?

        _____

36. How many tablets are needed to fill a prescription for 21 days for repaglinide 0.5 mg/tablet, one tablet three times a day?

        _____

37. How many capsules are needed to fill a prescription for 34 days for potassium chloride 10 mEq/capsule, one capsule four times a day?

        _____

38. How many capsules are needed to fill a prescription for three days for mefenamic acid 250 mg/capsule, one capsule four times a day?

        _____

39. How many tablets are needed to fill a prescription for 21 days for dipyridamole 50 mg/tablet, one tablet four times a day?

        _____

40. How many tablets are needed to fill a prescription for seven days for cyproheptadine 4 mg/tablet, one tablet three times a day?

        _____

CHAPTER 11

Percents

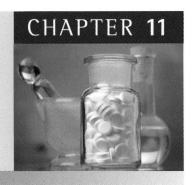

LEARNING OBJECTIVES

After completing this chapter, the student will be able to:

1 Explain the relationship between percents and decimals

2 Convert percents to decimals

3 Convert decimals to percents

KEY TERMS

Percent: per 100 or out of 100

Percent symbol: a way to write a fraction with a denominator of 100

THE TERM "PERCENT" means "per 100" or "out of 100."

The percent symbol (%) can be used as a way to write a fraction with a common denominator of 100.

EXAMPLE

20 out of every 100 equals 20%

EXAMPLE

5 out of every 100 equals 5%

EXAMPLE

15% = 15/100 = 0.15

Fifteen percent (15%) is the same as the fraction 15/100 and the decimal 0.15.

$\mathbb{R}$ CAPSULE   To convert a percent to decimal, just move the decimal point 2 places to the left and remove the "%" sign.

You can write percents as decimals by moving the decimal point two places to the left.

You can also write decimals as percents, by moving the decimal point two places to the right.

EXAMPLE

Express 27% as a decimal.

Because you can write a percent as a decimal by moving the decimal point two places to the left:

27% = 0.27

EXAMPLE

Express 0.85 as a percent.

Because you can write decimals as percents by moving the decimal point two places to the right:

.85 = 85%

EXAMPLE

Calculate 30% of 300.

1. Change 30% to a decimal by moving the decimal point two places to the left: 30% = 0.30

2. Then multiply: $0.30 \times 300 = 90$

Therefore, 30% of 300 is 90.

EXAMPLE

Write 6 out of 12 as a percent.

6 out of 12 = 0.5 = 50%

EXAMPLE

Find the value of n if n is 50% of 60.

$n = 0.5 \times 60 = 30$

EXAMPLE

Find the value of n if n is 150% of 24.

$n = 1.5 \times 24 = 36$

EXAMPLE

Find the value of n if n is 25% of 24.

$n = 0.25 \times 24 = 6$

EXAMPLE

Find the value of n if n is 110% of 40.

$n = 1.10 \times 40 = 44$

℞ CAPSULE   Percent strength for medication means the number of grams drug per 100 ml if in liquid or 100 grams if in solid.

EXAMPLE

Bactroban Nasal contains 2% mupirocin calcium. Express the strength as a decimal fraction.

2% = 2/100 = 0.02

PRACTICE PROBLEMS

STUDENT NAME _____

DATE _____ COURSE NUMBER _____

Express the following percents as decimals:

1. 33%   = _____   9. 75%   = _____

2. 24%   = _____   10. 83.32%   = _____

3. 33.3%   = _____   11. 66.66667% = _____

4. 50.5%   = _____   12. 18.5%   = _____

5. 20%   = _____   13. 1.3%   = _____

6. 47%   = _____   14. 0.25%   = _____

7. 93%   = _____   15. 0.125%   = _____

8. 32.5%   = _____

Express the following decimals as percents:

16. 0.2444   = _____   26. 0.52   = _____

17. 0.3   = _____   27. 0.4   = _____

18. 0.5   = _____   28. 0.65   = _____

19. 0.125   = _____   29. 0.025   = _____

20. 0.75   = _____   30. 0.035   = _____

21. 0.02   = _____   31. 0.055   = _____

22. 0.09   = _____   32. 0.004   = _____

23. 0.1   = _____   33. 1.10   = _____

24. 0.8   = _____   34. 1.75   = _____

25. 0.36   = _____   35. 2   = _____

Calculate the following:

36. 25% of 600   =   _____

37. 20% of 30   =   _____

38. 15% of 20   =   _____

39. 75% of 50   =   _____

40. 12.5% of 24   =   _____

41. 80% of 40   =   _____

42. 90% of 100   =   _____

43. 17% of 10   =   _____

44. 110% of 5   =   _____

45. 33% of 90   =   _____

46. 5% of 50   =   _____

47. 30% of 120   =   _____

48. 40% of 50   =   _____

49. 60% of 150   =   _____

50. 70% of 400   =   _____

Write the following expressions as percents:

51.   4 out of 5   =   _____

52.   2 out of 10   =   _____

53.   7 out of 8   =   _____

54.   15 out of 20   =   _____

55.   30 out of 35   =   _____

56.   85 out of 100   =   _____

57.   5 out of 8   =   _____

58.   3 out of 7   =   _____

59.   6 out of 20   =   _____

60.   12 out of 20   =   _____

61.   35 out of 40   =   _____

62.   40 out of 50   =   _____

63.   55 out of 100   =   _____

64.   80 out of 90   =   _____

65.   32 out of 64   =   _____

Find the value of n:

66.   If n is 20% of 50   n   =   _____

67.   If n is 35% of 24   n   =   _____

68.   If n is 60% of 8   n   =   _____

69. If n is 75% of 10   n   =   _____

70. If n is 80% of 15   n   =   _____

71. If n is 40% of 30   n   =   _____

72. If n is 50% of 100   n   =   _____

73. If n is 25% of 50   n   =   _____

74. If n is 30% of 90   n   =   _____

75. If n is 100% of 50   n   =   _____

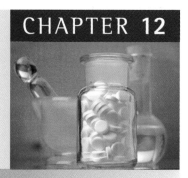

CHAPTER 12

Exponents and Scientific Notation

LEARNING OBJECTIVES

After completing this chapter, the student will be able to:

1 Define the term *exponent*

2 Define the term *scientific notation*

3 Express numbers given in exponential form as whole numbers

4 Express large numbers in scientific notation

KEY TERMS

Exponents: a shorthand way to show how many times a number is multiplied times itself

Scientific notation: expressing a number as a product of a number between 1 and 10 and a power of 10

EXPONENTS ARE A SHORTHAND WAY to show how many times a number is multiplied times itself. A number with an exponent is said to be "raised to the power" of that exponent.

EXAMPLE

$3^4 = 3 \times 3 \times 3 \times 3 = 81$

Any number raised to the zero power (except 0) equals 1.

(Ŗ CAPSULE) Any number raised to the power of zero equals 1.

EXAMPLE

$3^0 = 1$

Any number raised to the power of one equals itself.

EXAMPLE

$3^1 = 3$

EXAMPLE

$4^2 = 4 \times 4 = 16$

EXAMPLE

$5^3 = 5 \times 5 \times 5 = 125$

EXAMPLE

$10^3 = 10 \times 10 \times 10 = 1000$

Exponents of 10 are the most common form of exponents used in pharmacy calculations. As demonstrated in the previous example, the exponent tells us how many zeros follow.

EXAMPLE

$10^4 = 10,000$ and has four zeros

EXAMPLE

$10^2 = 100$ and has two zeros

For decimal fractions that are less than one, exponents are expressed as negative numbers. The number in the negative exponent tells us the number of decimal places.

EXAMPLE

$10^{-1} = 0.1$

EXAMPLE

$10^{-2} = 0.01$

EXAMPLE

$10^{-3} = 0.001$

Scientific Notation

Scientific notation is a short way of writing very long numbers. On a calculator, scientific notation is also known as E notation ("E" stands for "Exponent").

A number written in scientific notation is written as a product of a number between 1 and 10 and a power of 10.

EXAMPLE

Write 438,680,000 in scientific notation.

1. Change the number to a number between 1 and 10 by moving the decimal point 8 places to the left.

2. Multiply by 10 raised to the power of the number of places you had to move the decimal point.

$438,680,000 = 4.3868 \times 10^8$

On a calculator window, the base of 10 is not shown; the E means "10 raised to the following power."

EXAMPLE

Write the following numbers in scientific notation.

$434,000 = 4.34 \times 10^5$

$8,421,000 = 8.421 \times 10^6$

$23,412,000,000 = 2.3412 \times 10^{10}$

Decimal fractions that are less than one can also be expressed in scientific notation.

EXAMPLE

$0.34 = 3.4 \times 10^{-1}$

EXAMPLE

$0.021 = 2.1 \times 10^{-2}$

EXAMPLE

$0.00045 = 4.5 \times 10^{-4}$

PRACTICE PROBLEMS

STUDENT NAME _____

DATE _____ COURSE NUMBER _____

Express the following as numbers:

1. 2^3 = _____

2. 1^0 = _____

3. 1^1 = _____

4. 10^3 = _____

5. 3^{10} = _____

6. 6^6 = _____

7. 12^3 = _____

8. 10^5 = _____

9. 4^4 = _____

10. 5^5 = _____

11. 3^2 = _____

12. 4^3 = _____

13. 6^4 = _____

14. 7^2 = _____

15. 9^2 = _____

16. 10^2 = _____

17. 3^4 = _____

18. 4^7 = _____

19. 5^2 = _____

20. 6^3 = _____

Write the following numbers in scientific notation:

21. 12   = _____

22. 456   = _____

23. 5,309   = _____

24. 78,322   = _____

25. 104,043   = _____

26. 1,567,334   = _____

27. 0.12   = _____

28. 0.125   = _____

29. 0.0056   = _____

30. 2^3 = _____

31. 100   = _____

32. 1000   = _____

33. 5   = _____

34. 15   = _____

35. 30   = _____

36. 6,100   = _____

37. 712   = _____

38. 503   = _____

39. 35   = _____

40. 1,000,000   = _____

41. $0.032 = 3.2 \times 10^{-2}$ = _____

42. $0.157 = 1.57 \times 10^{-1}$ = _____

43. $0.0005 = 5 \times 10^{-4}$ = _____

44. $0.0257 = 2.57 \times 10^{-2}$ = _____

45. $1 = 1 \times 10^{0}$ = _____

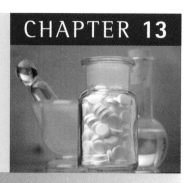

CHAPTER 13

Interpreting Prescriptions and Converting Household and Metric Measurements

LEARNING OBJECTIVES

After completing this chapter, the student will be able to:

1 Describe the metric system

2 Identify the standard metric units for length, weight, and volume

3 Define prefixes used in the metric system

4 Perform conversions between the metric system and household measurements

5 Perform conversions within the metric system

6 Interpret common pharmacy abbreviations

KEY TERMS

Metric system: system of measure based on the meter, liter, and gram

Gram (g): standard measure of weight in the metric system

Milliliter (ml or mL): common measure of volume in the metric system

Meter (m): standard measure of length in the metric system

Inscription: part of the prescription that provides information about the drug and amount

Signa (Sig): part of the prescription that provides the directions for use

DOCTORS ORDER MEDICATIONS for outpatients as prescriptions that are filled in pharmacies. Information is provided in prescriptions in a standard way (see Fig. 13-1). To perform necessary pharmacy calculations associated with filling prescriptions, two parts of the prescription are especially important: the *inscription* and the *signa*. The inscription gives the name of the medication and the amount to be dispensed. The signa provides instructions for use. Other elements of the prescription are required by law and are beyond the scope of this book. It is important for pharmacy technicians to know the common abbreviations that are used in prescriptions, and some common pharmacy abbreviations are listed in Table 13-1.

℞ CAPSULE   The inscription of a prescription provides the name of the medication and amount to dispense. The signa provides the directions for use.

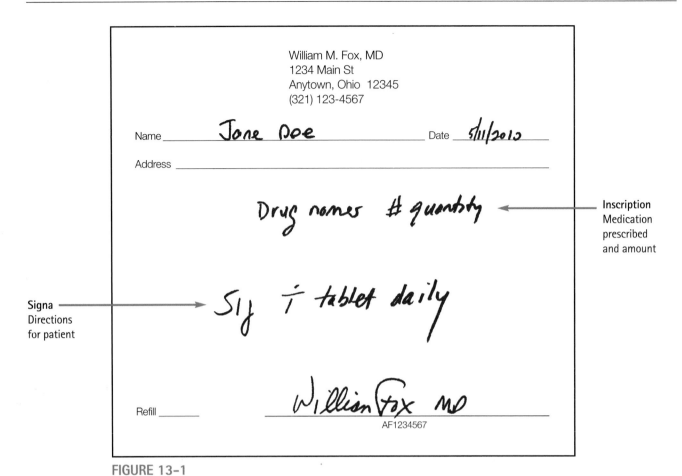

FIGURE 13-1

TABLE 13-1 **Common Pharmacy Abbreviations.** Abbreviations are commonly used in prescriptions to provide information that is necessary to prepare and administer the medication.

Abbreviation	Meaning	Abbreviation	Meaning
a.c.	before food	p.o.	by mouth
ad	to, up to	p.r.	by rectum
ad lib.	freely	p.r.n.	as needed
bib.	drink	qAM	each morning
b.i.d.	twice a day	q.d.	each day
$\bar{c}$	with	q.h.	each hour
gt or gtt	drop	q[2,3,4...]h	every [two, three, four, etc.] hours
h.s.	at bedtime	q.i.d.	four times a day
i.m.	into the muscle	qs	quantity sufficient*
i.v.	into the vein	Rx	take
non rep. or nr	do not repeat	$\bar{s}$	without
o.d.	right eye	s.l.	under the tongue
o.s.	left eye	stat.	immediately
o.u.	both eyes	t.i.d.	three times a day
p.c.	after food		* When qs is used in a compounded prescription, you should "add up" to the total amount indicated by qs with the appropriate ingredient.

The metric system is widely used in medicine. The strength of a medication is almost always given in metric units, most commonly the milligram (mg). For example, atenolol 50 mg tablets have 50 mg of the active ingredient (atenolol) in each tablet; however, if you weighed each tablet on a scale, you would find each tablet weighs much more than 50 mg (due to binders and fillers that are needed for the tablet to take form and hold together).

The metric system was developed in the late 1700s to replace a system with illogical units of measure with a rational system based on multiples of 10. The meter is the standard unit of length in the metric system and the length of the meter is based on the arc of the meridian from Barcelona, Spain, to Dunkirk, France. All metric units were derived from the meter. The gram is the standard measure of weight in the metric system (which is the weight of one cubic centimeter (cc) of water at its maximum density).

Greek prefixes were established for multiples of 10, ranging from pico- (one-trillionth) to tera- (one trillion) and including the more familiar micro- (one-millionth), milli- (one-thousandth), centi- (one-hundredth), and kilo- (one thousand). Thus, a kilogram equals 1000 grams, a millimeter 1/1000 of a meter.

One cubic centimeter (cc) is equal to one milliliter (ml). A milliliter is a measure of volume and there are 1000 milliliters in one liter.

Factor	Name	Symbol
10^9	giga	G
10^6	mega	M
10^3	kilo	k
10^2	hecto	h
10^1	deka	da
10^{-1}	deci	d
10^{-2}	centi	c
10^{-3}	milli	m
10^{-6}	micro	μ
10^{-9}	nano	n
10^{-12}	pico	p

EXAMPLE

How many centimeters (cm) are in one meter?

Because the prefix centi means 10^{-2}, there are 10^2 (or 100) centimeters in one meter.

EXAMPLE

How many milliliters (ml) are in one liter?

Because the prefix milli means 10^{-3}, there are 10^3 (or 1000) milliliters in one liter.

Converting Measurements

Medications are prepared by drug manufacturers according to the metric standards and measurements used in science. Pharmacies have an important duty to accurately convert metric measurements for the dose of medication to household measurements to ensure that patients get the correct dose of medication. The pharmacy label should provide information so the patient can read the directions on the prescription bottle, measure the correct dose of medication, and take the correct dose of medication.

Liquid medications taken by mouth are commonly dispensed in community pharmacies. Some but not all measuring spoons and measuring cups are labeled with both household and metric units. The directions are usually printed on the prescription label so the volume can be measured using household measuring devices such as measuring spoons, cups, etc.

Household Measure	Metric Equivalent
1 teaspoonful (tsp.)	5 ml
1 tablespoonful (Tbl.)	15 ml
1 fluid ounce (fl. oz.)	29.6 ml (often rounded to 30 ml)
1 pint (pt.)	473 ml (often rounded to 480 ml)
1 gallon (gal.)	3785 ml
1 pound (lb.)	454 gm

℞ CAPSULE   Liquid medications must be measured accurately and should be administered using a medicine dropper or medicine spoon. Household eating utensils do not provide accurate measurements.

The conversions between household and metric measurements can be done by carefully setting up proportions as fractions, then multiplying the fractions to get the correct answer.

℞ CAPSULE   **Important:** Always be sure you are using the correct conversion factors when setting up ratio and proportion or dimensional analysis equations.

EXAMPLE

Convert 2 tsp. to ml.

1. Start by setting up a dimensional analysis equation so the units you want in the final answer are in the numerator of the first fraction: 5 ml/1 tsp.

2. Set up the next fraction so the units of the numerator in the second fraction are the same as the units of the denominator in the first fraction (that is, so the units cancel when the fractions are multiplied): 2 tsp.

3. Multiply the fractions! Always be sure the numerator contains the units of the measuring device that you are using for your measurement: 5 ml/1 tsp. × 2 tsp. = 10 ml.

Important: Always double check your work to be sure the units cancel and the numerator contains the correct units. Also, be sure there was not an error using the calculator!

5 ml/1 tsp. × 2 tsp. = 10 ml

EXAMPLE

Convert 5 pints to milliliters.

1. Start by setting up a dimensional analysis equation so the units you want in the final answer are in the numerator of the first fraction: 473 ml/pint.

2. Set up the next fraction so the units of the numerator in the second fraction are the same as the units of the denominator in the first fraction (that is, so the units cancel when the fractions are multiplied): 5 pints.

3. Multiply the fractions.

$$\frac{473 \text{ ml}}{\text{pint}} \quad \bigg| \quad \frac{5 \text{ pints}}{} \quad = \quad 2,365 \text{ ml}$$

℞ CAPSULE   When calculating body weight from lbs to kg, use 2.2 lbs/kg.

EXAMPLE

A 66-lb child weighs how many kilograms?

1. Start by setting up a dimensional analysis equation so the units you want in the final answer are in the numerator of the first fraction: kg/2.2 lb.

2. Set up the next fraction so the units of the numerator in the second fraction are the same as the units of the denominator in the first fraction (that is, so the units cancel when the fractions are multiplied): 66 lb

3. Multiply the fractions.

$$\frac{\text{kg}}{2.2 \text{ lb}} \quad \bigg| \quad \frac{66 \text{ lbs}}{} \quad = \quad 30 \text{ kg}$$

EXAMPLE

If a prescription reads: 7.5 ml t.i.d., what is the dose in household units?

1 tsp./5 ml $\times$ 7.5 ml/dose = 1.5 tsp./dose

1. Start by setting up a dimensional analysis equation so the units you want in the final answer are in the numerator of the first fraction: 1 tsp./5 ml

2. Set up the next fraction so the units of the numerator in the second fraction are the same as the units of the denominator in the first fraction (that is, so the units cancel when the fractions are multiplied): 7.5 ml/dose

3. Multiply the fractions! Always be sure the numerator contains the units of the measuring device that you are using for your measurement: 1 tsp./5 ml $\times$ 7.5 ml/dose = 1.5 tsp./dose

Important: Again, remember to check your work!

EXAMPLE

If a prescription reads: Amoxicillin 250 mg/5 ml, dispense 150 ml, 375 mg t.i.d. $\times$ 5d, what is the dose in household units?

1 tsp./5 ml $\times$ 5 ml/250 mg $\times$ 375 mg/dose = 1.5 tsp./dose

EXAMPLE

If a medication is ordered 5 mg/kg/day and is administered once daily, what is the dose for a 150-pound patient?

$\dfrac{5 \text{ mg}}{\text{kg} \cdot \text{day}}$	$\dfrac{\text{kg}}{2.2 \text{ lbs}}$	$\dfrac{150 \text{ lbs}}{}$	= 340.9 mg/day

EXAMPLE

How many 50-ml bottles can be prepared from 1 L of simple syrup?

1. Start by setting up a dimensional analysis equation so that the units you want in the final answer are in the numerator of the first fraction: Bottle/50 ml

2. Set up the next fraction so that the units of the numerator in the second fraction are the same as the units of the denominator in the first fraction (that is, so that the units cancel when the fractions are multiplied): 1000 ml/L

3. Set up the next fraction so that the units of the numerator in the third fraction are the same as the units of the denominator in the second fraction (that is, so the units cancel when the fractions are multiplied): 1 L.

4. Multiply the fractions.

$\dfrac{\text{bottle}}{50 \text{ ml}}$	$\dfrac{1000 \text{ ml}}{\text{L}}$	$\dfrac{1 \text{ L}}{}$	= 20 bottles

PRACTICE PROBLEMS

Student Name _____

Date _____ Course Number _____

Convert the following:

1. 1/3 tsp.   = _____ ml

2. 3 tsp.   = _____ ml

3. 2 pints   = _____ ml

4. 1/2 lb.   = _____ gm

5. 3 quarts   = _____ ml   (*Hint:* 1 quart = 2 pints)

6. 1/2 tsp.   = _____ ml

7. 1 1/2 tsp.   = _____ ml

8. 3 gal.   = _____ ml

9. 3 tablespoonsful   = _____ ml

10. 2 fl. oz.   = _____ ml

11. 3 fl. oz.   = _____ ml

12. 3 pints   = _____ ml

13. 3 lbs.   = _____ gm

14. ml   = _____ tsp.

15. 45 ml   = _____ fl. oz.

16. 15 ml   = _____ tsp.   = _____ Tbl.

17. 2,365 ml   = _____ pints

18. 22,710 ml   = _____ gal.

19. 2 ml   = _____ tsp.

20. 20 ml   = _____ tsp.

21. 908 gm   = _____ lbs.

22. 45 ml   = _____ tsp.

23. 100 gm   = _____ lbs.

24. 3 Tbl.   = _____ ml

25. 5 fl. oz.   = _____ ml

26. 5 lbs.   = _____ kg

27. 1,135 gm   = _____ lbs.

28. 2 pt.   = _____ ml

29. 473 ml   = _____ pt.

30. 0.9 kg   = _____ lbs.

31. 9,080 gm   = _____ lbs.

32. 1000 mg   = _____ gm

33. 0.908 kg   = _____ lbs.

34. 3.785 liters = _____ gal.

35. 1.816 kg   = _____ lbs.

36. 1.75 tsp.   = _____ ml

37. 7.5 ml   = _____ Tbl.

38. 30 ml   = _____ tsp.

39. 60 ml   = _____ Tbl.

40. 88.8 ml   = _____ fl. oz.

41. If a prescription reads: Cefaclor 250 mg/5 ml, dispense 150 ml, 375 mg b.i.d. × 10d, what is the dose in teaspoonsful?   _____

42. If a prescription reads: Erythromycin 200 mg/5 ml, 200 mg t.i.d. × 5d, what is the dose in teaspoonsful?   _____

43. If the dose of a medication is 30 mg/kg/day in four divided doses, what is each dose for a 205-pound patient? (**Hints:** Use 2.2 lb/kg and note there are 4 doses per day.)   _____

44. If a prescription reads: Amoxicillin 50 mg/ml, dispense 30 ml, 62.5 mg t.i.d. × 5d, what is the dose in teaspoonsful?   _____

45. How many gallons of Coca Cola fountain syrup are needed to package 144 bottles of 120 ml per bottle?   _____

Converting Apothecary and Metric Measurements

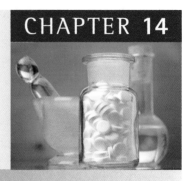

LEARNING OBJECTIVES

After completing this chapter, the student will be able to:

1 Describe the significance of apothecary measure in pharmacy

2 Perform conversion from apothecary to metric units

3 Perform conversion from metric to apothecary units

KEY TERMS

Apothecary system of measurement: a system of measurement associated with pharmaceuticals that uses ounces and grains

Metric system of measurement: a system of measurement associated with pharmaceuticals that uses grams, liters, and meters

SOME PRESCRIBERS ORDER MEDICATIONS using the apothecary system of measurement. The most commonly used apothecary measures are grains (to measure weight of solids) and drams (to measure volume of liquids).

Apothecary Measures

Apothecary Measure	Metric Equivalent
1 grain	64.8 mg (often rounded to 65 mg)
1 dram	5 ml
1 fl. oz.	29.6 ml (often rounded to 30 ml)
1 oz. (apothecary)	31 gm

> **℞ CAPSULE**   The weight of an apothecary ounce is different than the weight of an avoirdupois ounce. The avoirdupois ounce is used in commercial measures.

You can also perform the conversions between apothecary and household measurements by carefully setting up proportions as fractions, then multiplying the fractions to get the correct answer.

Important: Always be sure you are using the correct conversion factor when setting up ratio and proportion or dimensional analysis equations. Always double check your calculations!

EXAMPLE

Convert 129.6 mg to grains.

gr./64.8 mg × 129.6 mg = 2 gr.

EXAMPLE

If a prescription reads: Amoxicillin 250 mg/5 ml, dispense 150 ml, 1 dram t.i.d. × 10d, what is the dose in household units?

1 tsp./5 ml × 5 ml/1 dram × 1 dram/dose = 1 tsp./dose

EXAMPLE

If a prescription reads: aspirin 5 gr, dispense 100 tablets, 1 tablet q4-6h prn headache, what is the dose in milligrams?

64.8 mg/grain × 5 grains/tablet × 1 tablet/dose = 324 mg/dose

Important: Always be sure you are using the correct conversion factor when setting up ratio and proportions or dimensional analysis equations, and always double check your calculations!

EXAMPLE

A prescription calls for 93 g of hydrocortisone 2.5% cream. Convert 93 g to apothecary ounces.

1. Start by setting up a dimensional analysis equation so that the units you want in the final answer are in the numerator of the first fraction: oz./31 g.

2. Set up the next fraction so that the units of the numerator in the second fraction are the same as the units of the denominator in the first fraction (that is, so the units cancel when the fractions are multiplied): 93 g.

3. Multiply the fractions.

$$\frac{oz}{31\ g} \left| \begin{array}{c} 93\ g \end{array} \right. = 3\ oz$$

PRACTICE PROBLEMS

Student Name _____

Date _____ Course Number _____

Convert the following:

1. 3 gr.   = _____ mg

2. 1/2 gr.   = _____ mg

3. 3 drams   = _____ fl. oz.

4. 3 drams   = _____ ml

5. 1/2 dram   = _____ ml

6. 120 mg   = _____ gr.

7. 2 oz. (apothecary)   = _____ gm

8. 20 ml   = _____ drams

9. 30 ml   = _____ drams

10. 4 fl. oz.   =   _____ ml

11. 1/4 grain   =   _____ mg

12. 2 drams   =   _____ ml

13. 3 fl. oz.   =   _____ ml

14. 6 oz. (apothecary)   =   _____ gm

15. 2 grains   =   _____ mg

16. 5 drams   =   _____ ml

17. 2 fl. oz.   =   _____ ml

18. 12 oz. (apothecary) =   _____ gm

19. 97.2 mg   =   _____ grains

20. 60 ml   =   _____ drams

21. 59.2 ml   =   _____ fl. oz

22. 15.5 gm   =   _____ oz. (apothecary)

23. 194.4 mg   =   _____ grains

24. 120 ml   =   _____ drams

25. 44.4 ml   =   _____ fl. oz.

26. 46.5 gm   =   _____ oz. (apothecary)

27. 6 grain   =   _____ mg

28. 1/4 dram   =   _____ ml

29. 15 fl. oz.   =   _____ ml

30. 8 oz. (apothecary) =   _____ gm

31. If a prescription reads: Amoxicillin 250 mg/5 ml, dispense 150 ml, 1 dram t.i.d. $\times$ 10d, what is the dose in teaspoonsful?   _____

32. How many mg of phenobarbital are in one tablet of 2 grain phenobarbital?   _____

33. How many doses are in a 100 ml bottle of penicillin VK 250 mg/5 ml if each dose is 1/2 teaspoonful?   _____

34. If 100 tablets contain 40,000 mg of ibuprofen, how many grains are in 500 tablets?   _____

35. If a prescription reads: Theophylline Elixir 80 mg/15 ml, what is the dose in teaspoonsful if the required dose is 120 mg?   _____

CHAPTER 15

Converting Between the Different Temperature Scales

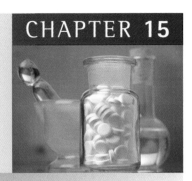

LEARNING OBJECTIVES

After completing this chapter, the student will be able to:

1 Explain the importance of proper storage temperatures for medications

2 Express an equation for converting Fahrenheit temperatures to Celsius

3 Perform calculations to convert temperature in degrees Fahrenheit to degrees Celsius

4 Perform calculations to convert temperature in degrees Celsius to degrees Fahrenheit

KEY TERMS

Fahrenheit: temperature scale in which the boiling point of water is at 212 degrees above the zero of the scale and the freezing point of water is at 32 degrees above the zero point of the scale and abbreviated by F

Celsius: temperature scale (also known as centigrade) in which the boiling point of water is at 100 degrees above the zero of the scale and the freezing point of water is at the zero point of the scale and abbreviated by C

THE TEMPERATURE FOR STORING MEDICATION is extremely important for the stability—and hence effectiveness—of the medication. The two common temperature scales used in pharmacy are Celsius and Fahrenheit. Usually storage requirements (including storage temperature) are listed in small print on the package label. The necessary temperature is usually given in both Celsius and Fahrenheit degrees, although not always. Therefore, you need to be able to convert between Celsius and Fahrenheit.

To convert to degrees Celsius from degrees Fahrenheit, use the following formula:

$T_c = (5/9)*(T_f - 32)$; T_c = temperature in degrees Celsius, T_f = temperature in degrees Fahrenheit

(In the formula, / means to divide, * means to multiply, − means subtract, + means to add and = means equals.)

EXAMPLE

Convert the Fahrenheit temperature of 98.6 degrees into degrees Celsius.

Using the above formula, first subtract 32 from the Fahrenheit temperature and get 66.6. Then, you multiply 66.6 by 5/9 and get 37 degrees Celsius.

The formula to convert a Celsius temperature into degrees Fahrenheit is:

Tf = (9/5)*Tc + 32; Tc = temperature in degrees Celsius, Tf = temperature in degrees Fahrenheit

(In the formula, / means to divide, * means to multiply, − means subtract, + means to add and = means equals.)

EXAMPLE

Convert the Celsius temperature of 100 degrees into degrees Fahrenheit.

Using the preceeding formula, you first multiply the Celsius temperature reading by 9/5 and get 180. Then, you add 32 to 180 and get 212 degrees Fahrenheit.

The temperature conversion formula can be simplified to:

9C = 5F − 160

℞ CAPSULE   Some people find the formula 9C = 5F − 160 is easier to use.

EXAMPLE

Use the formula 9C = 5F − 160 to convert the Celsius temperature of 100 degrees into Fahrenheit.

9(100) = 5F − 160

900 + 160 = 5F

1060 = 5F

212 = F

EXAMPLE

Use the formula 9C = 5F − 160 to convert 98.6 degrees Fahrenheit to degrees Celsius.

9C = 5(98.6) − 160

9C = 493 − 160

9C = 333

C = 37

PRACTICE PROBLEMS

STUDENT NAME _____

DATE _____   COURSE NUMBER _____

Convert the following (round your answer to the nearest whole degree):

1. 25 degrees Celsius   = _____ degrees Fahrenheit

2. 15 degrees Celsius   = _____ degrees Fahrenheit

3. 30 degrees Celsius   = _____ degrees Fahrenheit

4. 45 degrees Celsius   = _____ degrees Fahrenheit

5. 10 degrees Celsius   = _____ degrees Fahrenheit

6. 20 degrees Celsius   = _____ degrees Fahrenheit

7. 5 degrees Celsius   = _____ degrees Fahrenheit

8. 30 degrees Celsius   = _____ degrees Fahrenheit

9. 40 degrees Celsius   = _____ degrees Fahrenheit

10. 50 degrees Celsius   = _____ degrees Fahrenheit

11. 22 degrees Celsius   = _____ degrees Fahrenheit

12. 32 degrees Celsius   = _____ degrees Fahrenheit

13. 47 degrees Celsius   = _____ degrees Fahrenheit

14. 2 degrees Celsius   = _____ degrees Fahrenheit

15. 12 degrees Celsius   = _____ degrees Fahrenheit

16. –5 degrees Celsius   = _____ degrees Fahrenheit

17. –10 degrees Celsius   = _____ degrees Fahrenheit

18. 7 degrees Celsius   = _____ degrees Fahrenheit

19. 37 degrees Celsius   = _____ degrees Fahrenheit

20. 18 degrees Celsius   = _____ degrees Fahrenheit

21. 90 degrees Fahrenheit   = _____ degrees Celsius

22. 70 degrees Fahrenheit   = _____ degrees Celsius

23. 32 degrees Fahrenheit   = _____ degrees Celsius

24. 15 degrees Fahrenheit   = _____ degrees Celsius

25. 80 degrees Fahrenheit   = _____ degrees Celsius

26. 75 degrees Fahrenheit   = _____ degrees Celsius

27. 60 degrees Fahrenheit   = _____ degrees Celsius

28. 25 degrees Fahrenheit   = _____ degrees Celsius

29. 55 degrees Fahrenheit   = _____ degrees Celsius

30. 100 degrees Fahrenheit   = _____ degrees Celsius

31. 5 degrees Fahrenheit   = _____ degrees Celsius

32. 12 degrees Fahrenheit   = _____ degrees Celsius

33. 22 degrees Fahrenheit   = _____ degrees Celsius

34. 37 degrees Fahrenheit   = _____ degrees Celsius

35. 45 degrees Fahrenheit   = _____ degrees Celsius

36. 58 degrees Fahrenheit   = _____ degrees Celsius

37. 63 degrees Fahrenheit   = _____ degrees Celsius

38. 79 degrees Fahrenheit   = _____ degrees Celsius

39. 82 degrees Fahrenheit   = _____ degrees Celsius

40. 89 degrees Fahrenheit   = _____ degrees Celsius

Calculations for Community Pharmacy

 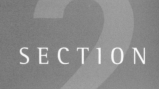

$2\% = 2 \text{ g}/100 \text{ ml} \quad Tf = 9/5 * Tc + 32 \quad 2.5 \text{ gm HC}/100 \text{ gm}$

In This Section

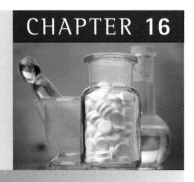

Calculations for Compounding

LEARNING OBJECTIVES

After completing this chapter, the student will be able to:

1 Explain why compounds are sometimes prescribed

2 Perform calculations to determine the amounts of ingredients needed to prepare compounds

KEY TERMS

Compound: a prescription prepared in the pharmacy for a product that is not commercially available

qs: abbreviation in the inscription of some compounds that means to "add up to" to the designated amount with the ingredient specified

COMPOUNDS ARE PREPARED in pharmacies for prescription orders that are not commercially available in the strength or form needed. Careful calculations are necessary to be sure the patient receives the proper dose of medication. You can also perform these calculations by carefully setting up ratio and proportion or dimensional analysis equations.

Important: Always be sure you are using the correct conversion factor when setting up ratio and proportion or dimensional analysis equations. Always double check your calculations!

EXAMPLE

How much hydrocortisone and how much Eucerin Cream must be weighed out to prepare the following compound?

Hydrocortisone 2.5% in Eucerin Cream

Dispense 60 gm

Sig: Apply sparingly b.i.d. prn

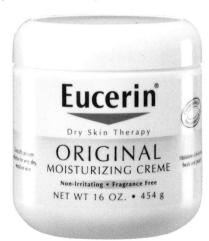

1. Calculate how much hydrocortisone is needed:

   2.5 gm HC/100 gm total × 60 gm total = 1.5 gm HC

2. Calculate how much Eucerin cream is needed:

Total weight = weight of hydrocortisone + weight of Eucerin cream

Using algebra, you can solve for the weight of the Eucerin cream:

Weight of Eucerin cream = Total weight − weight of hydrocortisone

Weight of Eucerin cream = 60 gm − 1.5 gm = 58.5 gm

EXAMPLE

If 100 gm of salicylic acid ointment contains 20 grams of salicylic acid, what is the percent strength of salicylic acid in the ointment?

20 gm salicylic acid/100 gm total ointment = 0.20 = 20%.

The inscription of the prescription for some compounds contains the abbreviation qs. This abbreviation is used in the inscription of some compounds when you need to "add up to" the stated amount with the particular ingredient.

EXAMPLE

Describe how to prepare the compound:

Rx   Maalox   15 ml
        Donnatal   15 ml
        Benadryl Elixir qs   120 ml

Use a graduate that measures 120 ml and first measure 15 ml of Maalox and place the Maalox in the graduate. Then add 15 ml of Donnatal and place the Donnatal in the graduate. Lastly, add enough Benadryl Elixir to the graduate so the total volume is 120 ml.

EXAMPLE

Determine how much Ora-Plus is needed to prepare 250 ml of calcium carbonate suspension using the following formula:

℞   Calcium carbonate   8 g
        Ora-Plus   35 ml
        Ora-Sweet   qs 100 ml

From the formula, we know 35 ml of OraPlus is needed for each 100 ml of the calcium carbonate suspension (35 ml OraPlus/100 ml calcium carbonate suspension).

We can use dimensional analysis to solve the problem.

$$\frac{35 \text{ ml Ora-Plus}}{100 \text{ ml calcium carbonate susp}} \times \frac{250 \text{ ml calcium carbonate susp}}{} = 87.5 \text{ ml OraPlus}$$

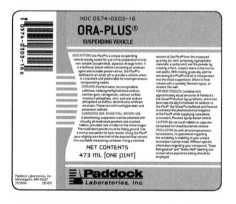

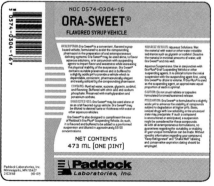

EXAMPLE

Determine how much glycerin is needed to prepare 500 glycerin
suppositories using the following formula:

R̸   Glycerin suppositories #100
       Glycerin   180 g
       Sodium stearate   17.8 g
       Purified water   9 ml

We can use dimensional analysis to solve the problem.

$$\frac{180 \text{ g glycerin}}{100 \text{ suppositories}} \quad \Big| \quad 500 \text{ suppositories} \quad = \quad 900 \text{ g glycerin}$$

Sometimes it is necessary to prepare products that have ingredients specified in percent strength. Usually the
ingredients are solids and sometimes the products are liquids, but other times the products are solids. When a
solid ingredient is expressed in percent strength of product when the product is a liquid, the percent strength tells
the number of grams of ingredient per 100 ml of product (ingredient g/100 ml product). When a solid ingredient
is expressed in percent strength of product when the product is a solid, the percent strength tells the number
of grams of ingredient per 100 g of product (ingredient g/100 g product). Chapter 29 is specifically devoted to
percentages.

EXAMPLE

Determine how much boric acid is needed to prepare 30 ml of boric acid 2% in 70% isopropyl alcohol.
(**Note:** 70% isopropyl alcohol is the solvent.)

We can use dimensional analysis to solve the problem.

$$\frac{2 \text{ g boric acid}}{100 \text{ ml prescription}} \quad \Big| \quad 30 \text{ ml prescription} \quad = \quad 0.6 \text{ g boric acid}$$

Reconstitution of Liquid Antibiotics for Oral Use

Most liquid antibiotics for oral use are shipped from the manufacturer in a powder form for reconstitution.
Distilled water is usually used for reconstitution of oral liquid antibiotics. In the powder form, the medications
have a longer shelf life than the liquid forms. Also, the powder forms can usually be stored at room temperature.
After reconstitution (adding the distilled water), the liquid antibiotics must often be stored in the refrigerator and
their shelf life is limited (usually 10 days to 35 days). Information about the shelf life of the reconstituted drug and
also how much distilled water must be added to get the desired concentration is printed on the manufacturer's
label.

Frequently, the manufacturer suggests that you add the distilled water in two-steps, so the liquid antibiotic is not
lumpy.

R̸ CAPSULE   Lumpy liquid antibiotics do not have uniform concentration of drug, and this can lead to variability in dosing.

EXAMPLE

To reconstitute a 150 ml bottle of amoxicillin for oral suspension 250 mg/5 ml, the manufacturer recommends 88 ml of distilled water is added in two divided portions. First, loosen the powder in the bottle, then add approximately 1/3 of the total volume of water and shake the suspension. After the powder is wet, add the remaining water. How much water should you add each time?

The first step is to calculate 1/3 of the total volume:

$1/3 \times 88 \text{ ml} = 29.3 \text{ ml}$ (For practical purposes you can round to 29 ml.)

The second step is to calculate the remaining amount of water:

Total volume = volume of 1st addition + volume of 2nd addition

Volume of 2nd addition = total volume − volume of 1st addition = 88 ml − 29 ml = 59 ml

Some antibiotics for injection are also supplied in powder form for reconstitution. Chapter 28 contains more information about calculations for powdered drugs for reconstitution.

PRACTICE
PROBLEMS

STUDENT NAME _____

DATE _____ COURSE NUMBER _____

1. How much (a) clindamycin phosphate (150 mg/ml) and how much (b) Cetaphil
   Lotion are needed to prepare the following compound?   (a) _____

   Clindamycin phosphate 600 mg in Cetaphil Lotion   (b) _____
   Dispense 60 ml
   Sig: Apply hs ud

2. A prescription is written for equal parts hydrocortisone cream 2.5% and Lamisil Cream,
   dispense 30 gm. How many grams of hydrocortisone 2.5% cream is needed to fill this
   prescription? What is the final concentration of hydrocortisone in the compound?   _____

3. A prescription is written for: Acyclovir 1200 mg, Silica gel. micronized 0.12 gm,
   Polyethylene glycol 3350 6.5 gm, Polyethylene glycol 400 15 ml. How many 200 mg
   capsules of acyclovir are needed to prepare this compound?   _____

4. A prescription is written for Allopurinol liquid 20 mg/ml in Ora-Plus:Ora-Sweet 1:1
   (label with a shelf-life of 60 days). How many tablets of allopurinol 100 mg are needed
   to prepare 150 ml?   _____

5. A prescription is written for Dilantin 5% in zinc oxide qs 120 gm. How many
   Dilantin 50 mg tablets are needed to prepare this compound?   _____

6. A prescription is written for ibuprofen 10% cream. How much ibuprofen powder
   is needed to prepare 30 grams of this compound?   _____

7. A prescription is written for Ichthammol Ointment 2 oz. How much ichthammol
   is needed to prepare 2 oz. if you are using the following formula: 100 grams of
   Ichthammol, 100 grams of Lanolin, 800 grams of Petrolatum, to make 1000 grams.   _____
   (*Hint:* Use 31 g = 1oz.)

8. A prescription is written for levothyroxine Na 25 mcg/ml, 100 ml to be compounded from crushed triturated with glycerin 40 ml (levitating agent and rinse for mortar and pestle) and water (q.s. 100 ml). This compound is stable for eight days when stored at 4 deg C. in amber bottles. How many 0.1 mg levothyroxine tablets are needed to prepare this compound?   _____

9. A prescription is written for Metoprolol tartrate 10 mg/ml Oral Liquid in a 50:50 mixture of Ora-Sweet:Ora Plus Vehicle q.s. 120 ml. How many Metoprolol tartrate 100 mg tablets are needed to prepare this compound?   _____

10. A prescription is written for Tetracycline HCl suspension 125 mg/5 ml compounded from capsules and a mixture of Ora-Plus 50% and Ora-Sweet 50%. How many capsules of Tetracycline 250 mg are needed to prepare 100 ml of this suspension?   _____

11. A prescription is written for salicylic acid 1%, menthol 1/4% in triamcinolone 0.1% cream. How much salicylic acid powder should be used if the prescription is for 240 gm?   _____

12. A prescription is written for a mouthwash containing 170 ml diphenhydramine elixir, 50 ml lidocaine viscous, 200 ml nystatin suspension, 52 ml of erythromycin ethyl succinate suspension, and 28 ml of cherry syrup to make 500 ml mouthwash. How much lidocaine viscous would be needed if you only need to prepare 100 ml of the mouthwash?   _____

13. You need to prepare 100 ml of hydrocortisone 2 mg/ml suspension. How many hydrocortisone 20 mg tablets will you need?   _____

14. You need to prepare 70 ml of lansoprazole 3 mg/ml suspension. How many lansoprazole 30 mg capsules will you need?   _____

15. You need to prepare 120 ml of potassium bromide 250 mg/ml. How much potassium bromide should you weigh?   _____

16. You need to prepare 150 ml of clonidine 0.1 mg/5 ml suspension. How many tablets of clonidine 0.2 mg/tablet will you need? _____

17. You need to prepare 300 ml of methylphenidate 10 mg/5 ml suspension. How many tablets of methylphenidate 20 mg/tablet will you need? _____

18. You need to prepare 50 ml of captopril 1 mg/ml suspension. How many tablets of captopril 50 mg/tablet will you need? _____

19. You need to prepare 45 ml of baclofen 10 mg/ml. How many tablets of baclofen 10 mg/tablet will you need? _____

20. You need to prepare 15 ml of amiptriptyline 20 mg/ml suspension. How many tablets of amitriptyline 50 mg/tablet will you need? _____

21. You need to prepare 90 ml of hydrochlorothiazide 10 mg/ml. How many tablets of hydrochlorothiazide 25 mg/tablet will you need? _____

22. You need to prepare 30 gm of salicylic acid 40% in petrolatum. How many gm of salicylic acid will you need? _____

23. You need to prepare 150 ml of metformin 100 mg/ml suspension. How many tablets of metformin 500 mg/tablet will you need? _____

24. You need to prepare a 150 ml of metronidazole 50 mg/5 ml suspension. How many tablets of metronidazole 250 mg/tablet will you need? _____

25. You need to prepare 60 ml of enalapril 1 mg/ml suspension. How many tablets of enalapril 10 mg/tablet will you need?   _____

26. You need to prepare 120 ml of amiodarone 5 mg/ml suspension. How many tablets of amiodarone 200 mg/tablet will you need?   _____

27. You are preparing hydrocortisone 2.4 g in 240 ml Lubriderm lotion. What is the percent strength of the hydrocortisone?   _____

28. You need to prepare 100 ml of celecoxib 100 mg/5 ml. How many capsules of 200 mg celecoxib/capsule will you need?   _____

29. You need 400 mg of promethazine to prepare 240 ml of PAC syrup. How many ml of promethazine 50 mg/ml will you need?   _____

30. You need to prepare 10 ml nitroglycerin 0.1 mg/ml from a stock vial of nitroglycerin 5 mg/ml diluted with normal saline. What volume of nitroglycerin 5 mg/ml will you need?   _____

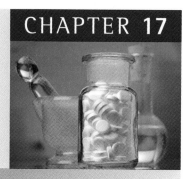

Calculations for Days Supply

CHAPTER 17

LEARNING OBJECTIVES

After completing this chapter, the student will be able to:

1 Explain why pharmacy technicians in community practice perform calculations for days supply

2 Explain why the same drug in the same quantity could last different amounts of time for different patients

3 Explain how to calculate days supply for prescriptions for tablets, capsules, and oral liquids

4 Explain how to estimate days supply for eyedrops, eardrops, creams, and ointments

5 Explain how to calculate days supply for metered-dose inhalers, specialized dosing packs, and insulin

6 Perform days supply calculations for prescriptions for tablets, capsules, oral liquids, insulin, and metered-dose inhalers

7 Estimate days supply for prescriptions for creams, ointments, eyedrops, and eardrops

KEY TERM

Days supply: a best estimate of how many days a prescription should last if taken as prescribed

INSURERS AND OTHER THIRD PARTIES that pay some or all of the price of a prescription have guidelines or dispensing limitations for how many days worth of medication they will pay for in a given time frame. The most common days supply limitation by third-party plans is a 34-day supply, although other days supply limitations exist, such as 30-day, 21-day, 14-day, etc.

Most prescribers write prescriptions with a different time frame in mind. Common prescribing time frames include 5 days, 1 week, 2 weeks, 1 month, 50 days, or 100 days.

Days Supply of Tablets, Liquids, Creams, Insulin, Inhalers, Eye Drops

Calculations for days supply should be the best estimate of how long a medication should last if it is used properly.

You can use ratio and proportion or dimensional analysis to solve calculations for days supply.

EXAMPLE

A prescription is written for Amoxicillin 250 mg capsules #30 i cap t.i.d. What is the days supply?

30 capsules × day/3 capsules = 10 days

EXAMPLE

A prescription is written for Amoxicillin 250 mg/5 ml 150 ml i tsp. t.i.d. What is the days supply?

150 ml × tsp./5 ml × dose/1 tsp. × day/3 doses = 10 days

Estimating days supply for some dosage forms, including creams and ointments, is not as straightforward. How long a product will last depends on the size of the area to be treated, and information about the size of the area to be treated is almost never written on prescriptions. In most cases, the amount of cream or ointment used per application is 500 mg − 1 g. To be safe, unless you know the size of the application area, use 1 g per application.

EXAMPLE

A prescription is written for Nystatin cream 15 gm apply sparingly twice a day. What is the days supply?

Calculations for creams are a little more tricky because you usually don't know how much cream will be used in a dose. The amount will depend on how large of an area is affected. The amount applied usually does not exceed 500 mg to 1 gram, so unless you know otherwise, use 1 gram for the amount of the dose.

15 gm × dose/1 gm × day/2 doses = 7.5 days (can round to 8 days)

> ℞ CAPSULE   Calculating days supply for creams, ointments, and gels is especially tricky because the size of the area for application is rarely provided with the prescription.

Prescriptions for insulin are often expressed in units per dose. However, the concentration of U-100 insulin is 100 units per milliliter (100 U/ml). To calculate days supply for U-100 insulin prescriptions, you will often need to use the conversion factor 100 U/ml.

EXAMPLE

A prescription is written for Humulin N U-100 insulin 10 ml 35 units daily. What is the days supply?

10 ml × 100 units/ml × dose/35 units ×
day/1 dose = 28.57 days (can round to 29 days)

> ℞ CAPSULE   The standard package size for insulin products is 10 ml.

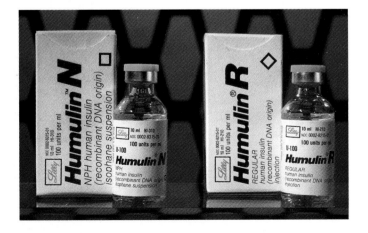

Prescriptions for metered-dose inhalers are often written in terms of the size of the containers. For metered-dose inhalers, the weight expressed for the container includes the weight of fillers in addition to the weight of the active drug. However, doses are usually expressed in terms of the number of metered doses per day or amount of the active ingredient per dose. To solve for days supply for metered-dose inhalers, you need to consider how many metered doses are in the container. When the dose is expressed in terms of the amount of active ingredient, you need to consider the amount of drug in each metered dose. Information about the amount of drug in each metered dose as well as the number of metered doses per container is provided with the package labeling.

EXAMPLE

A prescription is written for ProAir HFA Inhaler 8.5 gm 2 puffs q.i.d. What is the days supply?

To solve this problem, you should first read the manufacturer's label on the ProAir HFA Inhaler to determine how many metered doses are in each 8.5 gm container.

After reading the label, you determine each 8.5 gm container delivers 200 metered doses and you have enough information to solve the problem.

200 doses/1 container × day/8 doses = 25 days

Prescriptions for eyedrops and eardrops also require special care when calculating days supply. Doses are often expressed in terms of drops; however, for different products, the number of drops per ml can be different. To estimate days supply for eyedrops and eardrops you can estimate 20 drops/ml.

EXAMPLE

A prescription is written for Timolol 0.25% Opth.Sol. 5 ml i gtt ou q.d. What is the days supply?

To solve this problem you need to know how many drops are in 1 ml. The number of drops per ml is not a constant number and varies depending on physical properties of the solution or suspension as well as the size of the hole in the dropper. For most solutions or suspensions, there are 15–20 drops per ml. For the purpose of calculating days supply for third party claims, you can use 20 drops = 1 ml; however, this is only an estimation and *cannot* be used to calculate dosage.

5 ml/bottle × 20 drops/ml × day/2 drops × 50 days

> ℞ CAPSULE   For eyedrops and eardrops, 20 drops/ml provides a good estimate for calculating days supply.

Some medications come in specialized dosing packages. Examples are Medrol Dosepak and Decadron 5-12 Pak. For these medications, a different number of tablets is taken each day, and you may need to have the package or drug labeling in hand to determine the days supply.

EXAMPLE

What is the days supply for a Medrol Dosepak?

It is necessary to obtain more information about the product to solve the problem. From the manufacturer's packaging, we can determine that the package contains 21 tablets are taken in a tapering dose over a 6-day period, so the days supply is 6 days.

> ℞ CAPSULE   When calculating days supply for medications that come in specialized dosing packages, it is helpful to have the package in hand so you can read the directions that have been printed by the manufacturer.

PRACTICE PROBLEMS

STUDENT NAME _____

DATE _____ COURSE NUMBER _____

Calculate days supply for the following prescriptions:

1. Zantac 150 mg #60 one b.i.d. _____ days

2. Augmentin 500 mg #42 one t.i.d. _____ days

3. Prilosec 20 mg #50 one q.d. _____ days

4. Ampicillin 500 mg #40 one q.i.d. _____ days

5. Prozac 20 mg #60 one q.d. _____ days

6. Lamisil Cream 15 gm apply daily (*Hint:* Use 1 gm per application.) _____ days

7. Premarin 0.625 mg #100 one q.d. _____ days

8. Z-Pak 500 mg PO on first day of therapy, then 250 mg PO once daily for 4 days. Total cumulative dose 1.5 g (*Hint:* Check product labeling.) _____ days

9. Tylenol #3 Disp. #30 one-two q4-6h prn pain _____ days

10. Xanax 0.25 mg #30 one t.i.d. prn   _____ days

11. Terazol-7 Cream 45 gm
    Insert 1 applicatorful (5 gm) hs × 7d   _____ days

12. Lac-Hydrin 12% Lotion 150 ml
    Apply lotion twice daily to the affected skin areas and rub in thoroughly.
    (*Hint:* use 1–2 ml for amount used per application unless you know a larger
    area is being treated.)   _____ days

13. MetroGel Vaginal Gel 70 gm
    One applicatorful (37.5 mg of metronidazole/5 g cream)
    intravaginally b.i.d. × 5D   _____ days

14. Nizoral Cream 15 gm
    Apply to the affected and surrounding areas once daily for 2 weeks _____ days

15. Bactroban Oint. 15 gm
    Apply a small amount to the affected area t.i.d. × 1–2 weeks   _____ days

16. Humulin N U-100 10 ml
    35 U SQ daily   _____ days

17. Celebrex 200 mg #25
    1 cap q.d.   _____ days

18. Ultram 50 mg #20
     1–2 tab q4-6h prn pain   _____ days

19. Flonase 16 gm
     2 sprays per nostril (1 spray = 50 µg) once daily for a total daily dose of 200 µg
     (**Hint:** consider the 16 g container contains fillers and the 50 mcg (microgram)
     amount in the dose refers only to the active drug without fillers.) (From package
     labeling you can determine there are 120 metered doses per container.)   _____ days

20. Neosporin Opth. Ointment 3.5 gm
     Apply a thin strip (approx. = 1 cm ou q3-4 h × 7-10 d
     (**Hint:** 100 mg per eye per application is a useful estimate.)   _____ days

21. Ortho-TriCyclen 28
     One qd   _____ days

22. Viagra 50 mg #3
     50 mg PO prn not to exceed once daily   _____ days

23. HCTZ 25 mg/5 ml 150 ml
     12.5 mg q.d.   _____ days

24. Medrol Dosepak (#21 tablets)
     Take as labeled (**Hint:** see package, package insert or reference
     book for packaging information.)   _____ days

25. Tobradex Opth. Susp. 5 ml
    Instill 1–2 drops into the conjunctival sac os q4-6h (**Hint:** to estimate days
    supply for this problem, use two drops per dose in one eye six times per day
    [i.e., 12 drops per day].)   _____ days

26. Atrovent Inhalation Solution 0.02%
    2.5 ml × 25 vials 1 vial q.i.d.   _____ days

27. QVAR 80 mcg Inhaler 7.3 g 2 sprays (80 mcg/spray) p.o. b.i.d.
    (**Hint:** each inhaler contains 100 metered doses.)   _____ days

28. If a prescription is written for ibuprofen 600 mg, i tab q.i.d., what is the maximum
    quantity allowed if the third party plan has a 21-day dispensing limitation? _____

29. Atenolol 50 mg #100
    One q.d.   _____ days

30. Amoxicillin 250 mg #30
    One q8h   _____ days

31. Lisinopril 10 mg #30
    One daily   _____ days

32. Hydrochlorothiazide 25 mg #30
    One q.d.   _____ days

33. Furosemide Oral 20 mg po #25
    One q.d.

    _____ days

34. Alprazolam 0.5 mg #30
    One t.i.d.

    _____ days

35. Cephalexin 250 mg #28
    One q6h

    _____ days

36. Propoxyphene-N/APAP N-100 #60
    One q.i.d.

    _____ days

37. Metformin 500 mg #60
    One b.i.d.

    _____ days

38. Fluoxetine 20 mg #40
    One q.d.

    _____ days

39. Metoprolol Tartrate 50 mg #60
    One b.i.d.

    _____ days

40. Potassium Chloride 10 mEq #60
    One b.i.d.

    _____ days

41. Amoxicillin/Pot Clav 250 mg chewable #30
    One t.i.d.

    _____ days

42. Ranitidine HCl 150 mg #60
     One b.i.d.   _____ days

43. Amitriptyline 25 mg #30
     One h.s.   _____ days

44. Trimethoprim/Sulfa DS #20
     One b.i.d.   _____ days

45. Cyclobenzaprine 10 mg #30
     One t.i.d.   _____ days

46. Penicillin VK 500 mg #28
     One q.i.d.   _____ days

47. Tramadol 50 mg #36
     One q.i.d.   _____ days

48. Carisoprodol 350 mg #40
     One q.i.d.   _____ days

49. Verapamil SR 240 mg #30
     One q.d.   _____ days

CHAPTER 18

Adjusting Refills for Short-filled Prescriptions

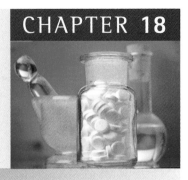

LEARNING OBJECTIVES

After completing this chapter, the student will be able to:

1 Describe how to adjust the fill quantity and refills to comply with limitations of third-party programs

2 Explain how refills are adjusted for insulin prescriptions

3 Identify medications that must be dispensed in original, unopened packages

THE AMOUNT OF MEDICATION a pharmacy can dispense to a patient is restricted first, by the prescriber's guidelines and second by the insurer's guidelines. Calculations are often needed to adjust first the quantity dispensed to comply with the insurer's guidelines, and then the number of refills allowed. Pharmacy technicians often need to accurately estimate how long a medication will last with inadequate guidelines. Estimating days supply is especially tricky when the dosage form is a lotion, cream, ointment, or inhalant.

When dispensing medications that come in handy convenience packages or dosage packages, such as methylprednisolone, estimate the days supply when you have the package in your hand so you can visually examine how it is packaged and read from the labeling or package insert how long the contents of the package should last. Usually, it is inappropriate to disrupt the packaging for medications that come in convenience packages or dosage packages, as well as nitroglycerin products that are packaged in glass containers.

> ℞ CAPSULE Third-party programs often have dispensing limitations that are less than the quantity of medication that has been prescribed.

EXAMPLE

A prescription is written for Dyazide #50 i cap q.d. + 3 refills. The insurance plan has a 34-day supply limitation. How many capsules can be dispensed using the insurance plan guidelines and how many refills are allowed with the adjusted quantity?

1. Calculate the total number of capsules allowed by the prescriber.

   50 capsules × 4 total fills (original fill + 3 refills) = 200 capsules

2. Using dimensional analysis, calculate the total number of fills of 34 capsules allowed:

   200 capsules × fill/34 capsules = 5.88 fills

The original prescription will have 4 additional refills of 34 capsules + 1 partial refill of 30 capsules.

EXAMPLE

A prescription is written for Rondec-DM Syrup 1 pint 1 teaspoonful h.s. + 1 refill. The insurance plan has a 34-day supply limitation. How many ml can be dispensed using the insurance plan guidelines and how many refills are allowed with the adjusted quantity?

1. Calculate the total volume allowed by the prescriber.

   1 pint × 2 fills (1 + 1 refill) = 2 pints

2. Convert to the metric quantity.

   2 pints × 473 ml/1 pint = 946 ml

3. Calculate the volume for a 34-day supply.

   5 ml/dose × 1 dose/day × 34 days/bottle = 170 ml

4. Calculate the number of refills.

   946 ml total × fill/170 ml = 5.56 total fills

Therefore, the answer is an original fill of 170 ml + 4 refills of 170 ml + a partial refill.

To calculate the amount of the partial refill:

.56 × 170 ml = 96 ml

You can check this:

946 ml − (5 fills × 170 ml per fill = 850 ml) = 96 ml

EXAMPLE

A prescription is written for Celebrex 200 mg capsules #100 i cap q.d. + no refills.
The insurance plan has a 21-day supply limitation. How many capsules can be dispensed using the insurance plan limitations, and how many refills are allowed with the adjusted quantity?

1. The total number of capsules allowed by the prescription is 100.

2. Using dimensional analysis, calculate the total number of fills of 21 capsules allowed:

   100 capsules × fill/21 capsules = 4.76 fills

3. The first fill of the prescription will have 21 capsules with three additional refills of 21 and one partial refill of 16 capsules.

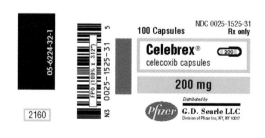

EXAMPLE

How many bottle(s) of insulin should be dispensed per fill if the prescription plan has a 34-day supply limit?

℞   Humulin R U-100 2 bottles

        Sig: 10 U t.i.d.

NR

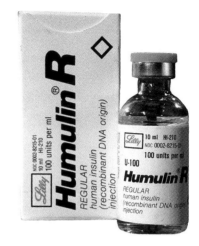

As we know, U-100 insulin contains 100 U/ml. A dimensional analysis setup can be used for this problem to determine how many days each bottle will last:

Day	Dose	100 U	10 ml		
3 doses	10 U	ml	bottle	=	33.3 days per bottle

Because 1020 units are used in a 34-day period, two bottles could be dispensed.

℞ CAPSULE   Although you can reduce the quantity to dispense for a prescription, you CANNOT exceed the prescribed quantity.

PRACTICE PROBLEMS

STUDENT NAME _____

DATE _____   COURSE NUMBER _____

Calculate the amount per fill allowable if a third-party plan covers a 34-day supply and adjust the refills:

1. Nitrolingual Pumpspray #3
    (200 sprays/container) 1–2 metered doses (400–800 μg) SL.
    May repeat q5 minutes up to a max. × 3 doses/15 min
    2 refills

    _____ qty   _____ refills   _____ partial

2. Atrovent Inhalation Solution 0.02%
    2.5 ml × 25 vials dispense
    10 boxes 1 vial q.i.d
    2 refills

    _____ qty   _____ refills   _____ partial

3. Humulin N U-100 Insulin 10 ml
    Dispense 4 bottles
    20 units daily
    3 refills

    _____ qty   _____ refills   _____ partial

4. Ultram 50 mg #120
    1 b.i.d.
    1 refill

    _____ qty   _____ refills   _____ partial

5. Timoptic 0.25% 10 ml
    Dispense 2 bottles 1 gtt ou q.d.
    3 refills (**Hint:** Use 20 drops/ml.) _____ qty   _____ refills   _____ partial

6. Betoptic 0.5% 10 ml
    Dispense 2 bottles
    1 gtt ou b.i.d.
    3 refill   _____ qty   _____ refills   _____ partial

7. Tobradex Opth. Susp. 5 ml
    1 gtt od q3-4h
    1 refill   _____ qty   _____ refills   _____ partial

8. Gentamicin Sulfate Opth. Ung. 3.5 gm
    Apply os b.i.d.
    1 refill (**Hint:** 3.5 gm = 1 tube) _____ qty   _____ refills   _____ partial

9. MS Contin 30 mg #120
    1 b.i.d.
    No refill
    (**Hint:** MS Contin is in
    DEA Schedule II.)   _____ qty   _____ refills   _____ partial

10. Cardizem CD 240 mg #120
    1 q.d.
    1 refill   _____ qty   _____ refills   _____ partial

11. Amitriptyline 25 mg #100
    1 h.s.
    1 refill   _____ qty   _____ refills   _____ partial

12. Methocarbamol 500 mg #240
    1000 mg p.o. q.i.d.
    1 refill   _____ qty   _____ refills   _____ partial

13. Nabumetone 500 mg #100
    1 g p.o. q.d.
    2 refills   _____ qty   _____ refills   _____ partial

14. Dicyclomine 20 mg #200
    20 mg p.o .q.i.d.
    1 refill   _____ qty   _____ refills   _____ partial

15. Chlorhexidine Gluconate 500 ml
    15 ml swish for 30 sec then spit b.i.d.
    3 refills   _____ qty   _____ refills   _____ partial

16. Albuterol Oral Liq 2 mg/5 ml 1 pint
    2 mg p.o. t.i.d.
    1 refill   _____ qty   _____ refills   _____ partial

17. Carbamazepine 200 mg #200
    1 q.i.d.
    2 refills   _____ qty   _____ refills   _____ partial

18. Indomethacin 25 mg #100
    1 b.i.d.
    2 refills   _____ qty   _____ refills   _____ partial

19. Hydroxychloroquine 200 mg #100
    2 q.d.
    2 refills   _____ qty   _____ refills   _____ partial

20. Digoxin 0.125 mg #100
    1 q.d.
    3 refills   _____ qty   _____ refills   _____ partial

21. Doxepin 150 mg #100
    One q.d. h.s.
    No refill   _____ qty   _____ refills   _____ partial

22. Mirtazapine 15 mg #50
    One q.d. h.s.
    No refill   _____ qty   _____ refills   _____ partial

23. Amiodarone 200 mg #100
    One q.d.
    No refill   _____ qty   _____ refills   _____ partial

24. Baclofen 20 mg #120
    One t.i.d.
    1 refill   _____ qty   _____ refills   _____ partial

25.   Benztropine 1 mg #100
       One b.i.d.
       1 refill   _____ qty   _____ refills   _____ partial

26.   Indapamide 1.25 mg #100
       One q.d.
       1 refill   _____ qty   _____ refills   _____ partial

27.   Labetalol 200 mg #100
       One b.i.d.
       1 refill   _____ qty   _____ refills   _____ partial

28.   Diltiazem SR 120 mg #100
       One b.i.d.
       2 refills   _____ qty   _____ refills   _____ partial

29.   Carbidopa/Levodopa 25/250 #100
       One b.i.d.
       2 refills   _____ qty   _____ refills   _____ partial

30.   Etodolac 400 mg #200
       One t.i.d.
       2 refills   _____ qty   _____ refills   _____ partial

CHAPTER 19

Calculations for Dispensing Fees, Co-pays, Difference Pricing

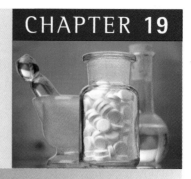

LEARNING OBJECTIVES

After completing this chapter, the student will be able to:

1 Define the term *dispensing fee*

2 Describe how co-pays are determined

3 Define the term *difference pricing*

4 Describe why some patients would be required to pay difference pricing

KEY TERMS

Dispensing fee: the amount a third-party program contracts to pay a pharmacy for the pharmacy's expenses associated with filling a prescription

Co-pay: the amount a patient pays for a prescription covered by a third-party program

Difference pricing: the amount in excess of the standard co-pay a patient must pay for a prescription when the third-party program only covers the cost of a generic and a brand name drug is dispensed

DISPENSING FEES ARE FEES that are determined by a contractual agreement between the third party and the pharmacy to pay for the expenses associated with dispensing each prescription (labor, equipment, rent, packaging, labeling, etc.).

Co-pays are determined by a contractual agreement between the third party and the patient and are usually determined by the insurer and/or employer providing the prescription drug benefits. Most co-pays are fixed dollar amounts and vary if a brand name or generic medication are dispensed. Some co-pays reflect a percent of the cost of the medication.

> ℞ CAPSULE   While some states have laws so patients can decline generic substitutions, most third-party plans only cover the price of the generic product. This means that in some cases, if the patient purchases the brand name product, the patient is responsible for the difference in cost between the brand and generic.

EXAMPLE

What is the co-pay for a prescription of Amoxicillin 250 mg #30 if the co-pay is 20% of the usual and customary price for the prescription and the usual and customary price for Amoxicillin 250 mg #30 is $8.49?

$0.2 \times \$8.49 = \$1.70$

Some insurance plans specify difference pricing must be used to calculate the co-pay of a prescription when a generic is available, but sometimes the patient refuses to get the generic. Although pharmacy technicians do not usually calculate difference pricing; it is helpful to understand difference pricing. The mathematical formula used to calculate the difference price varies among different third party plans and is specified in a contractual agreement. The difference price is usually determined by the sum of the co-pay amount plus the difference in cost between the brand and generic medication.

EXAMPLE

What is the co-pay for a prescription of Motrin 400 mg #20 if the brand name is specified by the patient, the co-pay amount is $5, the cost of Motrin 400 mg #20 is $3.74 and the cost of ibuprofen 400 mg #20 is $2.22?

$5	+	($3.74 − $2.22 = $1.52)	=	$6.52
standard		difference in cost between		difference
co-pay		brand and generic		price co-pay

EXAMPLE

How much will a pharmacy be reimbursed for a prescription if the third-party contract states the pharmacy will be reimbursed at 85% of AWP + $2.50 dispensing fee, and if the AWP for the prescription is $23.65?

0.85	× $23.65	= $20.10	+ $2.50		= $22.60
(fraction	AWP				amount
equal to			dispensing		pharmacy is
85%)			fee		reimbursed

EXAMPLE

What is the co-pay for a prescription of Glucophage 500 mg #60 if the brand name is specified by the patient, the co-pay amount is $15, the cost of Glucophage 500 mg #60 is $55.49 and the cost of metformin 500 mg #60 is $42.22?

$15 + ($55.49 − $42.22 = $13.27) = $28.27

EXAMPLE

What is the co-pay for a prescription of Ultram 50 mg # 30 if the brand name is specified by the patient, the co-pay amount is $25, the cost of Ultram 50 mg #30 is $49.25, and the cost of tramadol 50 mg #30 is $24.77?

$25 + ($49.25 − $24.77 = $24.48) = $49.48

PRACTICE PROBLEMS

STUDENT NAME _____

DATE _____ COURSE NUMBER _____

Determine the following co-pays if difference pricing is required by the third party plan.

1. What is the co-pay for a prescription of Hydrochlorothiazide 25 mg #30 if the co-pay is $5 and the usual and customary price for Hydrochlorothiazide 25 mg #30 is $6.09?   _____

2. What is the co-pay for a prescription of Micronase 5 mg #30 if the brand name is specified by the patient, the co-pay amount is $7, the cost of Micronase 5 mg #30 is $12.74, and the cost of Glyburide 5 mg #30 is $4.08?   _____

3. What is the co-pay for a prescription of Deltasone 5 mg #20 if the brand name is specified by the patient, the co-pay amount is $3, the cost of Deltasone 5 mg #20 is $2.08, and the cost of prednisone 5 mg #20 is $1.73?   _____

4. What is the co-pay for a prescription of Flagyl 250 mg #30 if the plan requires generic substitution and the co-pay is 20% of the usual and customary price? The usual and customary price for metronidazole 250 mg #30 is $12.08 and the usual and customary price for Flagyl 250 mg #30 is $34.77?   _____

5. What is the co-pay for a prescription of Aldactone 25 mg #30 if the co-pay is $5 for generic and $10 for brand names and the usual and customary price for spironolactone 25 mg #30 is $12.08?   _____

Calculate the difference price if the difference price is the sum of the co-pay amount + the difference in cost of the brand and generic.

6. What is the co-pay for a prescription of brand name Vicodin 5/500 #30 if there is no DAW on the prescription, but the patient wants to pay the difference pricing for the brand name? The co-pay amount is $5, the cost of Vicodin #30 is $18.05, and the cost of the generic #30 is $5.05.   _____

7. What is the co-pay for a prescription of brand name Tenormin 50 mg #30 if there is no DAW on the prescription, but the patient wants to pay the difference pricing for the brand name? The co-pay amount is $10, the cost of Tenormin 50 mg #30 is $35.40, and the cost of the generic #30 is $5.40.   _____

8. What is the co-pay for a prescription of brand name Zestril 5 mg #30 if there is no DAW on the prescription, but the patient wants to pay the difference pricing for the brand name? The co-pay amount is $15, the cost of Zestril 5 mg #30 is $26.40, and the cost of the generic #30 is $15.40.   _____

9. What is the co-pay for a prescription of brand name Xanax 0.5 mg #30 if there is no DAW on the prescription, but the patient wants to pay the difference pricing for the brand name? The co-pay amount is $5, the cost of Xanax 0.5 mg #30 is $26.40, and the cost of the generic #30 is $3.40.   _____

10. What is the co-pay for a prescription of brand name Keflex 500 mg #30 if there is no DAW on the prescription, but the patient wants to pay the difference pricing for the brand name? The co-pay amount is $15, the cost of Keflex 500 mg #30 is $84.40, and the cost of the generic is $2.40.

_____

11. What is the co-pay for a prescription for brand name Glucophage 500 mg #60 if there is no DAW on the prescription, but the patient wants to pay the difference pricing for the brand name? The co-pay amount is $20, the cost of Glucophage 500 mg #60 is $39.60, and the cost of the generic is $28.40.

_____

12. What is the co-pay for a prescription for brand name Prozac 20 mg #30 if there is no DAW on the prescription, but the patient wants to pay the difference pricing for the brand name? The co-pay amount is $15, the cost of Prozac 20 mg #30 is $85.40, and the cost of the generic is $25.70.

_____

13. What is the co-pay for a prescription for brand name Ativan 1 mg #30 if there is no DAW on the prescription, but the patient wants to pay the difference pricing for the brand name? The co-pay amount is $15, the cost of Ativan 1 mg #30 is $32.10, and the cost of the generic is $6.80.

_____

14. What is the co-pay for a prescription for brand name Augmentin 500 mg #30 if there is no DAW on the prescription, but the patient wants to pay the difference pricing for the brand name? The co-pay amount is $20, the cost of Augmentin 500 mg #30 is $108.20, and the cost of the generic is $88.10.

_____

15. What is the co-pay for a prescription for brand name Klonopin 1 mg #30 if there is no DAW on the prescription, but the patient wants to pay the difference pricing for the brand name. The co-pay amount is $15, the cost of Klonopin 1 mg #30 is $26.40, and the cost of the generic is $6.40.

_____

16. What is the co-pay for a prescription for brand name Bactrim DS #20 if there is no DAW on the prescription, but the patient wants to pay the difference pricing for the brand name. The co-pay amount is $20, the cost of Bactrim DS #20 is $38.40, and the cost of the generic is $3.90.

_____

17. What is the co-pay for a prescription for brand name Desyrel 100 mg #30 if there is no DAW on the prescription, but the patient wants to pay the difference pricing for the brand name. The co-pay amount is $25, the cost of Desyrel 100 mg #30 is $88.60, and the cost of the generic is $4.90.

_____

18. What is the co-pay for a prescription for brand name Flexeril 10 mg #30 if there is no DAW on the prescription, but the patient wants to pay the difference pricing for the brand name. The co-pay amount is $20, the cost of Flexeril 10 mg #30 is $28.40, and the cost of the generic is $3.90.

    _____

19. What is the co-pay for a prescription for Vasotec 10 mg #30 if there is no DAW on the prescription, but the patient wants to pay the difference pricing for the brand name. The co-pay amount is $15, the cost of Vasotec 10 mg #30 is $28.10, and the cost of the generic is $5.20.

    _____

20. What is the co-pay for a prescription for Valium 10 mg #30 if there is no DAW on the prescription, but the patient wants to pay the difference pricing for the brand name. The co-pay amount is $12, the cost of Valium 10 mg #30 is $63.20, and the cost of the generic is $5.30.

    _____

21. What is the co-pay for a prescription for Ultram 50 mg #30 if there is no DAW on the prescription, but the patient wants to pay the difference pricing for the brand name. The co-pay amount is $20, the cost of Ultram 50 mg #30 is $22.80, and the cost of the generic is $10.40.

    _____

22. What is the co-pay for a prescription for Soma 350 mg #30 if there is no DAW on the prescription, but the patient wants to pay the difference pricing for the brand name. The co-pay amount is $15, the cost of Soma 350 mg #30 is $108.10, and the cost of the generic is $5.40.   _____

23. What is the co-pay for a prescription for Calan SR 240 mg #30 if there is no DAW on the prescription, but the patient wants to pay the difference pricing for the brand name. The co-pay amount is $20, the cost of Calan SR 240 mg is $54.20, and the cost of the generic is $5.90.   _____

24. What is the co-pay for a prescription for Vibramycin 100 mg #20 if there is no DAW on the prescription, but the patient wants to pay the difference pricing for the brand name. The co-pay amount is $15, the cost of Vibramycin 100 mg #20 is $91.40, and the cost of the generic is $4.90.   _____

25. What is the co-pay for a prescription for Imdur 30 mg #30 if there is no DAW on the prescription, but the patient wants to pay the difference pricing for the brand name. The co-pay amount is $20, the cost of Imdur 30 mg #30 is $42.80, and the cost of the generic is $9.20.   _____

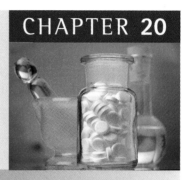

Calculations for Billing Compounds

LEARNING OBJECTIVES

After completing this chapter, the student will be able to:

1 Explain how third-party programs are billed for pharmacy compounds

2 Demonstrate an understanding that different third-party companies have different procedures for reimbursing pharmacies for compounded prescriptions

KEY TERM

Third-party programs: companies such as pharmacy benefit managers or insurers that are billed for prescriptions

CALCULATIONS FOR BILLING COMPOUNDS are determined by a contractual agreement by the third party and the pharmacy. The formula that should be used can vary among different third parties. Often, the formula is determined by the cost of the ingredients + a dispensing fee + a fee for the time it took to prepare the compound.

EXAMPLE

How much should an insurance company be billed for the following compound if the compound was prepared in 20 minutes and the dispensing fee is $3.25?

Hydrocortisone 2.5% in Eucerin Cream

Dispense 60 gm

Sig: Apply sparingly b.i.d. prn

1. Calculate how much hydrocortisone is needed:

   2.5 gm HC/100 gm total × 60 gm total = 1.5 gm HC

> ℞ CAPSULE   Some third-party programs have special requirements for entering compounded prescriptions into the computer and unique codes are needed for billing those third-party programs for compounded prescriptions.

2. Calculate the cost of the hydrocortisone (hydrocortisone comes in a 10 gm container that costs the pharmacy $31.25).

   1.5 gm HC × $31.25/10 gm HC = $4.69

3. Calculate how much Eucerin cream is needed:

   Total weight = weight of hydrocortisone + weight of Eucerin cream

   Using algebra, you can solve for the weight of the Eucerin cream

   Weight of Eucerin cream = total weight − weight of hydrocortisone

   Weight of Eucerin cream = 60 gm − 1.5 gm = 58.5 gm

4. Calculate the cost of the Eucerin if Eucerin comes from a 454 gm jar that costs the pharmacy $15.45:

   58.5 gm × $15.45/454 gm = $1.99

5. The amount to be billed is determined by adding the cost of the ingredients + the dispensing fee + the cost of the time to prepare the compound. You must next determine the cost of time to prepare the prescription:

   20 min × 1 hr/60 min × $35.00/hr = $11.67

   So the total amount of the prescription is:

$3.25	+	$4.69	+	$1.99	+	$11.67	=	$21.60
dispensing fee		cost of HC		cost of Eucerin		cost of time		total

How much should an insurance company be billed for the following compound if the compound was prepared in 10 minutes, the dispensing fee was $4.25, and the cost of ingredients was $3.75 using $50/hour to calculate cost of time?

R̸   Fluocinolone acetonide   10 mg

    Vegetable oil   qs 100 ml

1. Determine the cost of ingredients: $3.75.

2. The amount to be billed = cost of ingredients + dispensing fee + cost of time to prepare

   Amount to be billed = $3.75 + $4.25 + ($50/hr × hr/60 min × 10 min) = $16.33

PRACTICE PROBLEMS

STUDENT NAME_____

DATE _____ COURSE NUMBER _____

For the following problems use $35.00/hr to calculate the cost of time to prepare the prescription.

1. How much should an insurance company be billed for the following compound if the compound was prepared in 30 minutes and the dispensing fee is $3.25?   _____

    Ibuprofen 10% cream 30 grams

    Cost of ingredients = $12.47

2. How much should an insurance company be billed for the following compound if the compound was prepared in 10 minutes and the dispensing fee is $3.25?   _____

    Clindamycin phosphate 600 mg in Cetaphil Lotion
    Dispense 60 ml
    Sig: Apply hs ud

    Costs:
    Clindamycin phosphate 600 mg/ampule = $6.19
    Cetaphil Lotion 240 ml = $9.49

3. How much should an insurance company be billed for the following compound if the compound was prepared in 20 minutes and the dispensing fee is $3.25?   _____

    Hydrocortisone 2.5% in Eucerin Cream
    Dispense 60 gm
    Sig: Apply sparingly b.i.d. prn

    Costs:
    Hydrocortisone Powder 10 gm = $53.80
    Eucerin Cream 400 gm = $8.27

4. How much should an insurance company be billed for the following compound if the compound was prepared in 20 minutes and the dispensing fee is $3.25?

    Tetracycline HCl suspension 125 mg/5 ml compounded
    from capsules and a mixture of Ora-Plus 50% and
    Ora-Sweet 50% q.s. 200 ml

    Costs:
    Tetracycline 250 mg capsules = $0.23/capsule
    Ora-Plus 473 ml = $9.47
    Ora-Sweet 473 ml = $9.47

5. How much should an insurance company be billed for the the following compound if the compound was prepared in 20 minutes and the dispensing fee is $3.25?

    Metoprolol tartrate 10 mg/ml Oral Liquid in a 50:50 mixture
    of Ora-Sweet:Ora Plus Vehicle q.s. 120 ml

    Costs:
    Metoprolol tartrate 100 mg = $0.35/tablet
    Ora-Plus 473 ml = $9.47
    Ora-Sweet 473 ml = $9.47

6. How much should be charged for salicylic acid 1%, menthol 1/4% in triamcinolone 0.1% cream 60 gm if the dispensing fee is $4.25, the cost of ingredients is $8.40, and the compound was prepared in 20 minutes?

7. How much should be charged for menthol 1/4% in triamcinolone 0.1% cream 30 gm if the dispensing fee is $4.25, the cost of ingredients is $4.40, and the compound was prepared in 20 minutes?

8. How much should be charged for 170 ml diphenhydramine elixir, 50 ml lidocaine viscous, 200 ml nystatin suspension, 52 ml of erythromycin ethyl succinate suspension, and 28 ml of cherry syrup to make 500 ml if the dispensing fee is $4.25, the cost of ingredients is $18.40, and the compound was prepared in 20 minutes? _____

9. How much should be charged for 100 ml of hydrocortisone 2 mg/ml if the dispensing fee is $4.25, the cost of ingredients is $22.20, and the compound was prepared in 18 minutes? _____

10. How much should be charged for 70 ml of lansoprazole 3 mg/ml suspension if the dispensing fee is $4.25, the cost of ingredients is $38.14, and the compound was prepared in 15 minutes? _____

11. How much should be charged for 120 ml of potassium bromide 250 mg/ml if the dispensing fee is $4.25, the cost of ingredients is $6.25, and the compound was prepared in 10 minutes? _____

12. How much should be charged for 150 ml of clonidine 0.1 mg/5 ml suspension if the dispensing fee is $4.25, the cost of ingredients is $5.30, and the compound was prepared in 20 minutes? _____

13. How much should be charged for 300 ml of methylphenidate 10 mg/5 ml suspension if the dispensing fee is $4.25, the cost of ingredients is $36.20, and the compound was prepared in 15 minutes?   _____

14. How much should be charged for 50 ml of captopril 1 mg/ml suspension if the dispensing fee is $4.25, the cost of ingredients is $0.85, and the compound was prepared in 20 minutes?   _____

15. How much should be charged for 45 ml of baclofen 10 mg/ml if the dispensing fee is $4.25, the cost of ingredients is $7.25, and the compound was prepared in 20 minutes?   _____

16. How much should be charged for 15 ml of amiptriptyline 20 mg/ml suspension if the dispensing fee is $4.25, the cost of ingredients is $8.70, and the compound was prepared in 15 minutes?   _____

17. How much should be charged for 90 ml of hydrochlorothiazide 10 mg/ml if the dispensing fee is $4.25, the cost of ingredients is $4.20, and the compound was prepared in 15 minutes?   _____

18. How much should be charged for 30 gm of salicylic acid 40% in petrolatum if the dispensing fee is $4.25, the cost of ingredients is $11.40, and the compound was prepared in 20 minutes?   _____

19. How much should be charged for 150 ml of metformin 100 mg/ml suspension if the dispensing fee is $4.25, the cost of ingredients is $38.10, and the compound was prepared in 20 minutes?   _____

20. How much should be charged for 150 ml of metronidazole 50 mg/5 ml suspension if the dispensing fee is $4.25, the cost of ingredients is $16.20, and the compound was prepared in 20 minutes?   _____

21. How much should be charged for 60 ml of enalapril 1 mg/ml suspension if the dispensing fee is $4.25, the cost of ingredients is $19.10, and the compound was prepared in 20 minutes?   _____

22. How much should be charged for 120 ml of amiodarone 5 mg/ml suspension if the dispensing fee is $4.25, the cost of ingredients is $22.70, and the compound was prepared in 20 minutes?   _____

23. How much should be charged for hydrocortisone 2.4 g in 240 ml Lubriderm lotion
    if the dispensing fee is $4.25, the cost of ingredients is $21.50, and the compound
    was prepared in 20 minutes?   _____

24. How much should be charged for 100 ml of celecoxib 100 mg/5 ml if the dispensing fee
    is $4.25, the cost of ingredients is $21.15, and the compound was prepared in 15 minutes?   _____

25. How much should be charged for 240 ml PAC syrup if the dispensing fee is $4.25,
    the cost of ingredients is $32.20, and the compound was prepared in 20 minutes?   _____

Cash Register Calculations

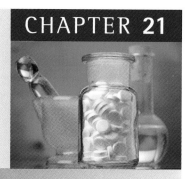

LEARNING OBJECTIVES

After completing this chapter, the student will be able to:

1 Describe how to make change for cash register transactions

2 Calculate how much change is due when a patient or customer pays with a different amount of money than the amount due

KEY TERMS

Cash payment: currency is used for payment of a prescription

Change: money returned when payment exceed the amount due

MOST CASH REGISTERS IN USE TODAY automatically calculate how much change is due when a customer pays. However, some cash registers do not automatically make this calculation, and sometimes patients or customers pay with a different amount of money than the amount entered into the cash register. Therefore, it is helpful to know how to do these calculations.

EXAMPLE

The price of a prescription is $15.45 and the patient pays with $20. How much change should you give to the patient?

To solve this problem, the change can be counted back to the patient in the following way:

1. 1 nickel makes $15.50

2. 2 quarters makes $16.00

3. 4 one dollar bills makes $20.00

The patient/customer is given $4.55.

> ℞ CAPSULE   In the retail setting it is important to be able to handle money. You must be able to give the correct change when you sell something. Being able to provide correct change fast and accurately makes you look smart and efficient.

EXAMPLE

The price of a prescription is $6.23 and the patient pays with $50. How much change is due in pennies, nickels, dimes, quarters, dollar bills, five dollar bills, ten dollar bills, and twenty dollar bills?

To solve the problem, the change can be counted back to the patient in the following way:

1. 2 pennies makes $6.25

2. 3 quarters makes $7.00

3. 3 one dollar bills makes $10.00

4. 2 twenty dollar bills makes $50.00

The patient/customer is given $43.77

EXAMPLE

The price of a prescription for Bactroban 2% ointment 22 grams is $74.50, and the patient pays with $80. Describe how change would be given.

To solve the problem, the change can be counted back to the patient in the following way:

1. 2 quarters makes $75.00

2. 1 $5 bill makes $80.00

EXAMPLE

The price of the prescription is $89.12, and the patient pays with $90. Describe how change would be given.

To solve the problem, the change can be counted back to the patient in the following way:

1. 3 pennies makes $89.15

2. 1 dime makes $89.25

3. 3 quarters makes $90

EXAMPLE

The price of the prescription is $75.45, and the patient pays with $100. Describe how change would be given.

1. 1 nickel makes $75.50

2. 2 quarters makes $76

3. 4 $1 bills makes $80

4. 1 $20 bill makes $100

PRACTICE PROBLEMS

STUDENT NAME _____

DATE _____ COURSE NUMBER _____

Calculate the amount of change due in pennies, nickels, dimes, quarters, dollar bills, five-dollar bills, ten-dollar bills, and twenty-dollar bills for the following transactions:

1. Amount of prescription: $16.41   Amount tendered: $50.00

    _____ pennies

    _____ nickels

    _____ dimes

    _____ quarters

    _____ one dollar bills

    _____ five dollar bills

    _____ ten dollar bills

    _____ twenty dollar bills

2. Amount of prescription: $35.22   Amount tendered: $50.00

    _____ pennies

    _____ nickels

    _____ dimes

    _____ quarters

    _____ one dollar bills

    _____ five dollar bills

    _____ ten dollar bills

3. Amount of prescription: $6.12   Amount tendered: $20.00

    _____ pennies

    _____ nickels

    _____ dimes

    _____ quarters

    _____ one dollar bills

    _____ five dollar bills

    _____ ten dollar bills

4. Amount of prescription: $42.50   Amount tendered: $50.00

_____ pennies

_____ nickels

_____ dimes

_____ quarters

_____ one dollar bills

_____ five dollar bills

5. Amount of prescription: $22.22   Amount tendered: $30.00

_____ pennies

_____ nickels

_____ dimes

_____ quarters

_____ one dollar bills

_____ five dollar bills

6. Amount of prescription: $26.25   Amount tendered: $40.00

_____ pennies

_____ nickels

_____ dimes

_____ quarters

_____ one dollar bills

_____ five dollar bills

_____ ten dollar bills

7. Amount of prescription: $1.03   Amount tendered: $50.00

_____ pennies

_____ nickels

_____ dimes

_____ quarters

_____ one dollar bills

_____ five dollar bills

_____ ten dollar bills

_____ twenty dollar bills

8. Amount of prescription: $44.41   Amount tendered: $60.00

_____ pennies

_____ nickels

_____ dimes

_____ quarters

_____ one dollar bills

_____ five dollar bills

_____ ten dollar bills

9. Amount of prescription: $9.80   Amount tendered: $100.00

_____ pennies

_____ nickels

_____ dimes

_____ quarters

_____ one dollar bills

_____ five dollar bills

_____ ten dollar bills

_____ twenty dollar bills

10. Amount of prescription: $12.06   Amount tendered: $50.06

_____ pennies

_____ nickels

_____ dimes

_____ quarters

_____ one dollar bills

_____ five dollar bills

_____ ten dollar bills

_____ twenty dollar bills

11. Amount of prescription: $63.12   Amount tendered: $70.00

_____ pennies

_____ nickels

_____ dimes

_____ quarters

_____ one dollar bills

_____ five dollar bills

_____ ten dollar bills

_____ twenty dollar bills

12. Amount of prescription: $41.59   Amount tendered: $50.00

_____ pennies

_____ nickels

_____ dimes

_____ quarters

_____ one dollar bills

_____ five dollar bills

_____ ten dollar bills

_____ twenty dollar bills

13. Amount of prescription: $163.12   Amount tendered: $180.00

_____ pennies

_____ nickels

_____ dimes

_____ quarters

_____ one dollar bills

_____ five dollar bills

_____ ten dollar bills

_____ twenty dollar bills

14. Amount of prescription: $23.55   Amount tendered: $40.00

_____ pennies

_____ nickels

_____ dimes

_____ quarters

_____ one dollar bills

_____ five dollar bills

_____ ten dollar bills

_____ twenty dollar bills

15. Amount of prescription: $89.04   Amount tendered: $100.04

_____ pennies

_____ nickels

_____ dimes

_____ quarters

_____ one dollar bills

_____ five dollar bills

_____ ten dollar bills

_____ twenty dollar bills

16. Amount of prescription: $113.42   Amount tendered: $200.00

_____ pennies

_____ nickels

_____ dimes

_____ quarters

_____ one dollar bills

_____ five dollar bills

_____ ten dollar bills

_____ twenty dollar bills

17. Amount of prescription: $3.82   Amount tendered: $20.00

_____ pennies

_____ nickels

_____ dimes

_____ quarters

_____ one dollar bills

_____ five dollar bills

_____ ten dollar bills

_____ twenty dollar bills

18. Amount of prescription: $18.99   Amount tendered: $50.00

_____ pennies

_____ nickels

_____ dimes

_____ quarters

_____ one dollar bills

_____ five dollar bill

_____ ten dollar bills

_____ twenty dollar bills

19. Amount of prescription: $198.89   Amount tendered: $200.00

_____ pennies

_____ nickels

_____ dimes

_____ quarters

_____ one dollar bills

_____ five dollar bills

_____ ten dollar bills

_____ twenty dollar bills

20. Amount of prescription: $311.44   Amount tendered: $320.00

_____ pennies

_____ nickels

_____ dimes

_____ quarters

_____ one dollar bills

_____ five dollar bills

_____ ten dollar bills

_____ twenty dollar bills

21. Amount of prescription: $5.05   Amount tendered: $20.05

_____ pennies

_____ nickels

_____ dimes

_____ quarters

_____ one dollar bills

_____ five dollar bills

_____ ten dollar bills

_____ twenty dollar bills

22. Amount of prescription: $59.98   Amount tendered: $60.03

_____ pennies

_____ nickels

_____ dimes

_____ quarters

_____ one dollar bills

_____ five dollar bills

_____ ten dollar bills

_____ twenty dollar bills

23.   Amount of prescription: $115.52   Amount tendered: $120.02   _____ pennies

_____ nickels

_____ dimes

_____ quarters

_____ one dollar bills

_____ five dollar bills

_____ ten dollar bills

_____ twenty dollar bills

24.   Amount of prescription: $10.98   Amount tendered: $20.00   _____ pennies

_____ nickels

_____ dimes

_____ quarters

_____ one dollar bills

_____ five dollar bills

_____ ten dollar bills

_____ twenty dollar bills

25.   Amount of prescription: $71.51   Amount tendered: $80.01   _____ pennies

_____ nickels

_____ dimes

_____ quarters

_____ one dollar bills

_____ five dollar bills

_____ ten dollar bills

_____ twenty dollar bills

26.   Amount of prescription: $49.53   Amount tendered: $50.03

_____ pennies

_____ nickels

_____ dimes

_____ quarters

_____ one dollar bills

_____ five dollar bills

_____ ten dollar bills

_____ twenty dollar bills

27.   Amount of prescription: $101.37   Amount tendered: $120.00

_____ pennies

_____ nickels

_____ dimes

_____ quarters

_____ one dollar bills

_____ five dollar bills

_____ ten dollar bills

_____ twenty dollar bills

28.   Amount of prescription: $57.84   Amount tendered: $60.00

_____ pennies

_____ nickels

_____ dimes

_____ quarters

_____ one dollar bills

_____ five dollar bills

_____ ten dollar bills

_____ twenty dollar bills

29. Amount of prescription: $143.32   Amount tendered: $160.00   _____ pennies

_____ nickels

_____ dimes

_____ quarters

_____ one dollar bills

_____ five dollar bills

_____ ten dollar bills

_____ twenty dollar bills

30. Amount of prescription: $48.45   Amount tendered: $100.00   _____ pennies

_____ nickels

_____ dimes

_____ quarters

_____ one dollar bills

_____ five dollar bills

_____ ten dollar bills

_____ twenty dollar bills

Usual and Customary Prices

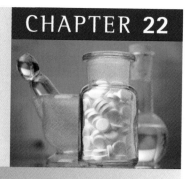

LEARNING OBJECTIVES

After completing this chapter, the student will be able to:

1 Define *usual and customary price* for a prescription
2 Describe how usual and customary price can be determined

KEY TERM

Usual and customary price (U&C): the standard price for a prescription when the patient pays without third-party coverage

THE USUAL AND CUSTOMARY PRICE (U&C) is the price charged to patients who pay cash for prescriptions. U&C prices are usually determined in the corporate offices. For some new medications and medications that are rarely used, U&C prices are sometimes determined in the pharmacy using a formula provided by corporate management. This formula may already be programmed into the pharmacy computer system so the U&C price can be determined automatically when a prescription is filled.

EXAMPLE

If prescription prices are determined using the following formula:

AWP + professional fee = selling price of prescription

The professional fee is determined using a chart such as the following:

AWP	Professional Fee
Less than $20.00	$4.00
$20.01 − $50.00	$5.00
Greater than $50.01	$6.00

℞ CAPSULE In the retail setting, professional fees and pricing formulas are determined by the employer.

EXAMPLE

If the AWP for 30 capsules of amoxicillin 250 mg is $3.50, what will be the selling price of the prescription?

Since the AWP for the prescription is less than $20.00, the professional fee is $4.00.

Using the formula:

AWP + professional fee = selling price of prescription

$3.50 + $4.00 = $7.50

Some pharmacies sell certain medications at a price lower than the acquisition cost. Therefore, the usual and customary price may be less than the average wholesale price (AWP) or less than the acquisition cost. Many third-party plans reimburse the pharmacy based on the lowest amount: AWP, acquisition cost, or U&C, since the third parties do not want to pay more for a prescription than the patient would pay in cash.

EXAMPLE

If the AWP for Zithromax 250 mg Z-Pak is $47.72, what will be the selling price of the prescription if the professional fee is $5.00 (*Note:* Z-Pak contains six tablets)?

$47.72 + $5.00 = $52.72

EXAMPLE

If the AWP for Accolate 20 mg #30 is $40.20, what will be the selling price of the prescription if the professional fee is $5.00?

$40.20 + $5.00 = $45.20

EXAMPLE

If the AWP for Avondia 8 mg #30 is $165.90, what will be the selling price of the prescription if the professional fee is $6.00?

$165.90 = $6.00 = $171.90

EXAMPLE

If the AWP for Prozac 20 mg #30 is $115.50, what will be the selling price of the prescription if the professional fee is $6.00?

$115.50 + $6.00 = $121.50

EXAMPLE

A prescription is filled for one 10 ml bottle of Humulin N U-100 insulin. The AWP is $33.75. The U&C price for one bottle of Humulin N U-100 insulin is $43.00.

If the pharmacy has an agreement with the third-party plan for reimbursement of 87% AWP or 100% U&C (whichever is less) + a $4.50 dispensing fee, what will be the total amount of the third-party claim?

First, determine the lowest cost basis for calculation of the third-party claim.

.87 × $33.75 = $29.36

$29.36 (87% AWP) is less than $43.00 (U&C); therefore, calculation of the third-party claim will be based on the lower amount.

The total third-party claim will be $29.36 + $4.50 = $33.86.

PRACTICE PROBLEMS

STUDENT NAME_____

DATE _____ COURSE NUMBER _____

Calculate the retail price of the following prescriptions using the formula AWP + professional fee = retail price of prescription if the professional fee is determined using the following chart:

AWP	Professional Fee
less than $20.00	$4.00
$20.01 − $50.00	$5.00
Greater than $50.01	$6.00

1. Verapamil SR Tabs #30 AWP/100 $120.85 retail price _____

   36.25   41.25

2. Glyburide 5 mg Tabs #30 AWP/1000 $440.05 retail price _____

3. Dexamethasone 4 mg Tabs #12 AWP/100 $58.40 retail price _____

   11.00 $\frac{58.40}{100} \times \frac{12}{(12)} = 7.00 + 4.00$

4. Danazol 200 mg Caps #100 AWP/100 $306.38 retail price _____

5. Doxepin 150 mg Caps #30 AWP/100 $66.50 retail price _____

6. Tetracycline 250 mg Caps #28 AWP/1000 $52.43 retail price _____

7. Docusate Calcium 240 mg Caps #30 AWP/100 $9.90 retail price _____

8.   Amantadine Syrup 4 oz. AWP/PINT $61.51   retail price _____

9.   Fluocinolone Cream 0.025% 15 Gm AWP/15 GM $3.05   retail price _____

10. Acebutolol 400 mg Caps #60 AWP/100 $121.51   retail price _____

11. Guanabenz 4 mg Tabs #30 AWP/100 $66.20   retail price _____

12. Hydrocortisone Valerate Cream 0.2% 45 GM AWP/45 GM $28.14   retail price _____

13. Hydrocodone/APAP 5/500 #30 AWP/100 $14.80   retail price _____

14. Atenolol 50 mg #30 AWP/100 $5.20   retail price _____

15. Amoxicillin 250 mg #30 AWP/100 $2.20   retail price _____

16. Lisinopril 10 mg #30 AWP/100 $14.40   retail price _____

17. Hydrochlorothiazide 25 mg #30 AWP/100 $4.80   retail price _____

18. Furosemide Oral 20 mg #30 AWP/100 $5.40   retail price _____

19. ProAir HFA 8.5 gr AWP/8.5 gm $40.98   retail price _____

20. Alprazolam 0.25 mg #30 AWP/100 $5.60   retail price _____

21. Cephalexin 500 mg #40 AWP/100 $19.60   retail price _____

22. Triamterene w/HCTZ 37.5 mg/25 mg AWP/100 $12.10   retail price _____

If the pharmacy has an agreement with the third party plan for reimbursement of 87% AWP or 100% U&C (whichever is less) + a $3.50 dispensing fee, what will be the total amount of the third party claim for the following prescriptions?

23. Verapamil SR Tabs #30 AWP/100 $120.85 retail price/30 $40.20   amount of claim _____

24. Danazol 200 mg Caps #100 AWP/100 $306.38 retail price/30 $95.39   amount of claim _____

25. Doxepin 150 mg Caps #30 AWP/100 $66.50 retail price/30 $28.60   amount of claim _____

26. Tetracycline 250 mg Caps #28 AWP/1000 $52.43 retail price/28 $6.99   amount of claim _____

27. Amantadine Syrup 4 oz. AWP/PINT $61.51 retail price/4 oz. $28.60   amount of claim _____

28. Amitriptyline 50 mg #90 AWP/100 $5.40 retail price/90 $8.99   amount of claim _____

29. Clonazepam 1 mg #30 AWP/100 $15.20 retail price/90 $22.59   amount of claim _____

30. Warfarin 5 mg #30 AWP/100 $29.90 retail price/30 $15.99   amount of claim _____

31. Trimethoprim/Sulfa #20 AWP/100 $12.30 retail price/30 $8.99   amount of claim _____

32. Trazodone 50 mg #30 AWP/100 $11.40 retail price/30 $8.99   amount of claim _____

33. Cyclobenzaprine 10 mg #30 AWP/100 $14.30 retail price/30 $8.49   amount of claim _____

34. Enalapril 20 mg #30 AWP/100 $13.90 retail price/30 $11.99   amount of claim _____

35. Carisoprodol 350 mg #30 AWP/100 $24.80 retail price/30 $17.99   amount of claim _____

36. Verapamil SR 180 mg #30 AWP/100 $15.60 retail price/30 $12.99   amount of claim _____

37. Doxycycline 100 mg #20 AWP/100 $33.40 retail price/20 $12.99   amount of claim _____

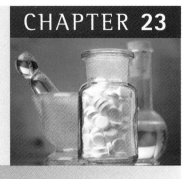

CHAPTER 23

Discounts

LEARNING OBJECTIVES

After completing this chapter, the student will be able to:

1 Describe when pharmacies may offer discounts

2 Demonstrate the ability to calculate 5% discounts and 10% discounts

KEY TERM

Discount: a reduction made from the regular price

PHARMACIES SOMETIMES GIVE a 5% or 10% discount on the price of prescriptions to certain patients such as senior citizens who are not participating in third party programs. State pharmacy regulations or third party contractual agreements may prohibit discounting prescriptions that are covered by third party programs. Sometimes, the discount is restricted to prescriptions purchased on certain days of the week.

> ℞ CAPSULE   A discount is simply a reduction in price. Sometimes discounts are in percent, such as a 10% discount, and then you need to do a calculation to find the price reduction.

EXAMPLE

A senior citizen is paying for a prescription for amoxicillin 250 mg #30. The usual and customary price is $8.49; however this patient qualifies for a 10% discount. How much will the patient pay?

$$\$8.49 - 10\% \,(\$8.49) = \$8.49 - (0.1)(\$8.49) = \$8.49 - \$0.85 = \$7.64$$

EXAMPLE

Calculate the amount the patient would pay if the patient qualifies for a 5% discount and the retail price is $74.27.

$$\$74.27 - 5\%(\$74.27) = \$74.27 - (0.05)(\$74.27) = \$74.27 - \$3.71 = \$70.56$$

EXAMPLE

Calculate the amount the patient would pay if the patient qualifies for a 5% discount and the retail price is $121.45.

$121.45 − 5%($121.45) = $121.45 − (0.05)($121.45) = $121.45 − $6.07 = $115.38

EXAMPLE

Calculate the amount the patient would pay if the patient qualifies for a 10% discount and the retail price is $195.20.

$195.20 − 10%($195.20) = $195.20 − (0.1)($195.20) = $195.20 − $19.52 = $175.68

PRACTICE PROBLEMS

STUDENT NAME _____

DATE _____ COURSE NUMBER _____

Calculate how much the patient will pay for the following prescriptions if the patient qualifies for a 5% discount:

1. Retail price for prescription is $4.99   after 5% discount the patient pays _____

2. Retail price for prescription is $12.47   after 5% discount the patient pays _____

3. Retail price for prescription is $35.20   after 5% discount the patient pays _____

4. Retail price for prescription is $89.90   after 5% discount the patient pays _____

5. Retail price for prescription is $120.47   after 5% discount the patient pays _____

6. Retail prices for prescriptions are $5.60 + $27.50   after 5% discount the patient pays _____

7. Retail prices for prescriptions are $22.10 + $68.50   after 5% discount the patient pays _____

8. Retail prices for prescriptions are $21.60 + $153.50   after 5% discount the patient pays _____

9. Retail prices for prescriptions are $5.60 + $67.12   after 5% discount the patient pays _____

10. Retail prices for prescriptions are $97.60 + $127.30   after 5% discount the patient pays _____

11. Retail price for prescriptions are
$5.40 + $9.90 + $15.20

after 5% discount the patient pays _____

12. Retail price for prescriptions are
$15.20 + $8.30 + $95.20

after 5% discount the patient pays _____

13. Retail price for prescriptions are
$42.15 + $18.25 + $195.20

after 5% discount the patient pays _____

14. Retail price for prescriptions are
$65.20 + $78.20 + $19.10

after 5% discount the patient pays _____

15. Retail price for prescriptions are
$95.45 + $18.30 + $75.20

after 5% discount the patient pays _____

16. Retail price for prescriptions are
$121.20 + $118.30 + $135.20

after 5% discount the patient pays _____

17. Retail price for prescriptions are
$83.19 + $118.23 + $45.79

after 5% discount the patient pays _____

18. Retail price for prescriptions are
$111.11 + $88.30 + $35.27

after 5% discount the patient pays _____

19. Retail price for prescriptions are
$66.30 + $118.15 + $125.20

after 5% discount the patient pays _____

20. Retail price for prescriptions are
$118.20 + $183.20 + $192.50

after 5% discount the patient pays _____

Calculate how much the patient will pay for the following prescriptions if the patient qualifies for a 10% discount:

21. Retail price for prescription is $4.99   after 10% discount the patient pays _____

22. Retail price for prescription is $12.47   after 10% discount the patient pays _____

23. Retail price for prescription is $35.20   after 10% discount the patient pays _____

24. Retail price for prescription is $89.90   after 10% discount the patient pays _____

25. Retail price for prescription is $120.47   after 10% discount the patient pays _____

26. Retail prices for prescriptions are $5.60 + $27.50   after 10% discount the patient pays _____

27. Retail prices for prescriptions are $22.10 + $68.50   after 10% discount the patient pays _____

28. Retail prices for prescriptions are $21.60 + $153.50   after 10% discount the patient pays _____

29. Retail prices for prescriptions are $5.60 + $67.12   after 10% discount the patient pays _____

30. Retail prices for prescriptions are $97.60 + $127.30   after 10% discount the patient pays _____

31. Retail price for prescriptions are
     $123.52 + $118.33 + $95.27   after 10% discount the patient pays _____

32. Retail price for prescriptions are
    $15.29 + $118.30 + $9.20

    after 10% discount the patient pays _____

33. Retail price for prescriptions are
    $135.20 + $82.30 + $135.30

    after 10% discount the patient pays _____

34. Retail price for prescriptions are
    $125.24 + $18.23 + $93.23

    after 10% discount the patient pays _____

35. Retail price for prescriptions are
    $15.32 + $8.35 + $65.29

    after 10% discount the patient pays _____

36. Retail price for prescriptions are
    $115.30 + $18.40 + $15.32

    after 10% discount the patient pays _____

37. Retail price for prescriptions are
    $125.10 + $18.70 + $90.10

    after 10% discount the patient pays _____

38. Retail price for prescriptions are
    $19.90 + $18.80 + $15.50

    after 10% discount the patient pays _____

39. Retail price for prescriptions are
    $15.66 + $112.30 + $155.23

    after 10% discount the patient pays _____

40. Retail price for prescriptions are
    $15.55 + $8.88 + $95.60

    after 10% discount the patient pays _____

Gross and Net Profits

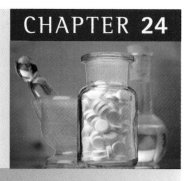

GROSS PROFIT IS THE DIFFERENCE between the selling price and acquisition price of an item, while net profit is the difference between the selling price and all associated costs (including the acquisition price).

Gross Profit

The gross profit is the difference between the selling price and the acquisition cost. For cash prescriptions, the selling price is the usual and customary price for prescriptions paid by cash customers. For third party prescriptions, the selling price is determined by a contractual agreement for prescriptions paid by third parties. To calculate gross profit, there is no consideration for any of the expenses associated with filling the prescription.

Gross profit = selling price − acquisition cost

The gross profit can be expressed as a percent.

EXAMPLE:

A prescription for amoxicillin 250 mg #30 has a usual and customary price of $8.49. The acquisition cost of amoxicillin 250 mg #30 is $2.02. What is the gross profit?

Gross profit = selling price − acquisition cost

Gross profit = $8.49 − $2.02 = $6.47

Net Profit

The net profit is the difference between the selling price of the prescription and the sum of all the costs associated with filling the prescription. All the costs associated with filling the prescription include the cost of the medication, the cost of the container, the cost of the label, the cost of the bag, the cost of the labor to dispense the prescription, a portion of the rent, etc. For practical purposes, all the other costs can be grouped together and considered as a dispensing fee. Since the costs associated with operation of a pharmacy vary, the dispensing fee can vary.

Net profit = selling price − acquisition cost − dispensing fee

or

Net profit = gross profit − dispensing fee

Net profit can also be expressed as a percent.

> ℞ CAPSULE   The net profit is equal to the gross profit minus the costs associated with filling the prescription.

EXAMPLE

A prescription for amoxicillin 250 mg #30 has a usual and customary price of $8.49. The acquisition cost of amoxicillin 250 mg #30 is $2.02. What is the net profit if the dispensing fee/professional fee is $5.50?

Net profit = selling price − acquisition cost − dispensing fee

Net profit = $8.49 − $2.02 − $5.50 = $0.97

EXAMPLE

If the dispensing fee is $6.00, calculate the gross profit and net profit for the following prescription if the acquisition cost is $77.20 and the selling price is $92.99.

Tamiflu 75 mg #10

Gross profit = selling price − acquisition cost

Gross profit = $92.99 − $77.20 = $15.79

Net profit = selling price − acquisition cost − dispensing fee

Net profit = $92.99 − $77.20 − $6.00 = $9.79

EXAMPLE

If the dispensing fee is $6.00, calculate the gross profit and net profit for the following prescription if the acquisition cost is $294.00 and the selling price is $353.13.

Sporanox 100 mg #30

Gross profit = selling price − acquisition cost

Gross profit = $353.13 − $294.00 = $59.13

Net profit = selling price − acquisition cost − dispensing fee

Net profit = $353.13 − $294.00 − $6.00 = $53.13

EXAMPLE

If the dispensing fee is $6.00, calculate the gross profit and net profit for the following prescription if the acquisition cost is $134.70 and the selling price is $222.67.

Gross profit = selling price − acquisition cost

Gross profit = $222.67 − $134.70 = $87.97

Net profit = selling price − acquisition cost − dispensing fee

Net profit = $222.67 − $134.70 − $6.00 − $81.97

PRACTICE PROBLEMS

STUDENT NAME_____

DATE _____ COURSE NUMBER _____

Use this table to determine the dispensing/professional fee:

AWP	Dispensing/Professional Fee
less than $20.00	$4.00
$20.01 − $50.00	$5.00
Greater than $50.01	$6.00

then calculate the gross profit and the net profit for the following prescriptions:

1. Zocor 5 mg, 60 tablets, acquisition cost = $85.47, AWP = $106.84, selling price = $109.93

   Gross profit = _____

   Net profit   = _____

2. Prilosec 20 mg, 30 cap., acquisition cost = $99.20, AWP = $108.90, selling price = $116.38

   Gross profit = _____

   Net profit   = _____

3. Norvasc 5 mg, 90 tablets, acquisition cost = $97.92, AWP = $125.66, selling price = $117.82

   Gross profit = _____

   Net profit   = _____

4. Procardia XL 30 mg, 100 tablets, acquisition cost = $105.05 AWP = $131.31, selling price = $134.36

   Gross profit = _____

   Net profit   = _____

5. Vasotec 10 mg, 100 tablets, acquisition cost = $85.56, AWP = $102.94, selling price = $109.19

   Gross profit = _____

   Net profit   = _____

6. Relafen 500 mg, 100 tablets, acquisition cost = $88.88, AWP = $111.10, selling price = $120.27

   Gross profit = _____

   Net profit   = _____

7. Zoloft 50 mg, 100 tablets, acquisition cost = $172.44, AWP = $215.55, selling price = $226.50

     Gross profit = _____

     Net profit   = _____

8. Fosamax 10 mg, 30 tablets, acquisition cost = $50.91, AWP = $51.88, selling price = $57.62

     Gross profit = _____

     Net profit   = _____

9. Cardizem CD 240 mg, 90 tablets, acquisition cost = $154.10, AWP = $165.42, selling price = $179.69

     Gross profit = _____

     Net profit   = _____

10. Ticlid 250 mg, 60 tablets, acquisition cost = $99.44, AWP = $108.90, selling price = $122.07

     Gross profit = _____

     Net profit   = _____

11. Atenolol 50 mg, 90 tablets, acquisition cost = $5.80, AWP = $9.80, selling price = $15.99

     Gross profit = _____

     Net profit   = _____

12. Amoxicillin 500 mg 90 capsules, acquisition cost = $7.80, AWP = $12.80, selling price = $18.99

     Gross profit = _____

     Net profit   = _____

13. Lisinopril 20 mg 90 tablets, acquisition cost = $35.80, AWP = $42.80, selling price = $45.99

     Gross profit = _____

     Net profit   = _____

14. Hydrochlorothiazide 50 mg 90 tablets, acquisition cost = $1.80, AWP = $4.80, selling price = $10.99

     Gross profit = _____

     Net profit   = _____

15. Furosemide 20 mg 90 tablets, acquisition cost = $3.20,
    AWP = $7.90, selling price = $10.99

    Gross profit = _____

    Net profit   = _____

16. ProAir HFA 8.5 gm, acquisition cost = $37.50,
    AWP = $40.98, selling price = $43.50

    Gross profit = _____

    Net profit   = _____

17. Alprazolam 1 mg 90 tablets, acquisition cost = $4.90,
    AWP = $9.80, selling price = $17.99

    Gross profit = _____

    Net profit   = _____

18. Prednisone 10 mg 90 tablets, acquisition cost = $2.80,
    AWP = $8.60, selling price = $12.99

    Gross profit = _____

    Net profit   = _____

19. Metformin 500 mg 60 tablets, acquisition cost = $25.80,
    AWP = $32.80, selling price = $36.99

    Gross profit = _____

    Net profit   = _____

20. Fluoxetine 20 mg 30 capsules, acquisition cost = $25.20,
    AWP = $39.80, selling price = $45.99

    Gross profit = _____

    Net profit   = _____

21. Metoprolol 50 mg 60 tablets, acquisition cost = $5.20,
    AWP = $8.80, selling price = $11.99

    Gross profit = _____

    Net profit   = _____

22. Lorazepam 1 mg 30 tablets, acquisition cost = $8.80,
    AWP = $9.80, selling price = $15.99

    Gross profit = _____

    Net profit   = _____

23. Amitriptyline 25 mg 90 tablets, acquisition cost = $5.80, AWP = $7.80, selling price = $12.99

Gross profit = _____

Net profit   = _____

24. Enalapril 5 mg 90 tablets, acquisition cost = $15.80, AWP = $19.80, selling price = $25.99

Gross profit = _____

Net profit   = _____

25. Tramadol 50 mg 30 tablets, acquisition cost = $12.80, AWP = $15.80, selling price = $22.99

Gross profit = _____

Net profit   = _____

26. Carisoprodol 350 mg 30 tablets, acquisition cost = $7.85, AWP = $9.93, selling price = $15.99

Gross profit = _____

Net profit   = _____

27. Verapamil SR 120 mg 90 tablets, acquisition cost = $32.80, AWP = $35.80, selling price = $45.99

Gross profit = _____

Net profit   = _____

28. Doxycycline 100 mg 20 capsules, acquisition cost = $5.20, AWP = $6.70, selling price = $10.99

Gross profit = _____

Net profit   = _____

29. Isosorbide Mononitrate 60 mg CR 30 tablets, acquisition cost = $25.80, AWP = $29.90, selling price = $37.99

Gross profit = _____

Net profit   = _____

30. Glyburide micronized 3 mg 60 tablets, acquisition cost = $12.80, AWP = $19.80, selling price = $25.99

Gross profit = _____

Net profit   = _____

CHAPTER 25

Inventory Control

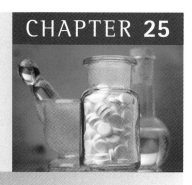

LEARNING OBJECTIVES

After completing this chapter, the student will be able to:

1 Explain why inventory affects the bottom line

2 Explain how minimum/maximum level inventory systems work

3 Calculate reorder quantities using minimum/maximum inventory levels

KEY TERMS

Inventory: a list of the goods on hand

Inventory control: supervising the supply and accessibility of the goods on hand to ensure adequate supply without excessive oversupply

MOST PHARMACIES MUST BORROW MONEY and pay interest on the borrowed money in order to keep an adequate supply of medications on the shelf with which to fill all anticipated prescriptions. The amount paid toward the interest for borrowing money to keep drugs on the shelf affects the operating expenses and therefore affects the net profit or "bottom line."

Ideally, pharmacies could have all drugs on the shelf at all times; but this is practically impossible due to the high cost of medications. Although pharmacy technicians are usually not involved in securing loans for the pharmacy, they should have some appreciation for the expenses associated with maintaining an inventory and the significance of inventory control.

The expenses associated with borrowing money can be calculated using the following equation:

$$B = A(1 + r/n)^{NT} - P[(1 + r/n)^{NT} - 1]/[(1 + r/n) - 1]$$

where

B = balance after t (or T) years
A = amount borrowed
n or N = number of payments per year
P = amount paid per payment
r = annual percentage rate (APR)

If an amount A is borrowed and will be repaid by n repayments per year, each of an amount P, interest will accumulate at an annual percentage rate of r, and this interest will compound n times a year (along with each payment). Installments will be of amount P until the original amount and any accumulated interest is repaid. This equation gives the amount B that will be repaid after t years.

Rather than working through this equation to calculate the expenses associated with borrowing money, computer programs or tables are usually used. Therefore, it is not practical for a pharmacy technician to solve problems using this equation, but it is important to have an appreciation for the expenses associated with maintaining an inventory of prescription drugs.

As the amount of money paid for interest on borrowed money increases, profits decrease. Therefore, in order to maximize profits, the pharmacy inventory should be as low as possible while having enough medication in stock to fill prescriptions.

Computerized methods for inventory control are evolving; however, human intervention is necessary for the computerized methods to be effective. Computerized methods can be based on minimum/maximum level inventory systems. In minimum/maximum level inventory systems, drugs are reordered up to the maximum inventory level when the minimum inventory level is reached.

The maximum inventory level − # bottle(s) on hand = order quantity (# bottles)

℞ CAPSULE   When using minimum/maximum inventory systems for ordering, the minimum/maximum control specifies the point at which an item should be reordered (minimum stocking level) and a reorder quantity ceiling (maximum stocking level).

EXAMPLE

Amoxicillin 250 mg capsules are stocked in 500 ct. bottles. The acquisition cost to the pharmacy for each 500 ct. bottle is $55.50. The shelf label indicates the minimum/maximum inventory level for amoxicillin 250 mg 500 ct. is 2/4. There is only a partial bottle on the shelf. Should this medication be reordered? If so, how many bottles should you order?

Answer: Since the minimum shelf quantity is 2 and there is only 1 bottle on the shelf, yes the medication should be reordered. The medication should be reordered up to the maximum shelf quantity.

The maximum inventory level − # bottle(s) on hand = order quantity (bottle(s))

4 bottles (maximum) − 1 bottle (on hand) = 3 bottles (order)

EXAMPLE

Determine the reorder quantities for the following medication using information from the minimum/maximum inventory levels on the shelf labels and the on-hand quantities.

Humulin N U100
Minimum/maximum inventory level   10/40
On hand   8

Because there are fewer than 10 bottles on the shelf, it is appropriate to reorder. To determine the number of bottles to order, subtract the number of bottles on hand from the maximum inventory level.

Maximum inventory level − number of bottles on hand = reorder quantity

40 − 8 = 32

EXAMPLE

Determine the reorder quantities for the following medication using information from the minimum/maximum inventory levels on the shelf labels and the on-hand quantities.

Flonase 0.05% Nasal Spray
Minimum/maximum inventory level   2/6
On hand   3

Because there are more than two bottles on the shelf, it is not appropriate to reorder at this time.

EXAMPLE

Determine the reorder quantities for the following medication using information from the minimum/maximum inventory levels on the shelf labels and the on-hand quantities.

Hyzaar 100-25 Tab
Minimum/maximum inventory level   2/3
On hand   1

Because there are fewer than two bottles on the shelf, it is appropriate to reorder. To determine the number of bottles to order, subtract the number of bottles on hand from the maximum inventory level.

Maximum inventory level − number of bottles on hand = reorder quantity

3 − 1 = 2

PRACTICE PROBLEMS

STUDENT NAME _____

DATE _____   COURSE NUMBER _____

Determine the reorder quantities for the following medication using information from the minimum/maximum inventory levels on the shelf labels and the on-hand quantities:

1. Ambien 5 mg
    minimum/maximum inventory level   1/2
    on hand   1   reorder quantity _____

2. Terazol-3
    minimum/maximum inventory level   6/12
    on hand   4   reorder quantity _____

3. Pepcid 20 mg
    minimum/maximum inventory level   2/5
    on hand   4   reorder quantity _____

4. Prozac 20 mg
    minimum/maximum inventory level   6/12
    on hand   1   reorder quantity _____

5. Nitrostat 0.4 mg 4 × 25s
    minimum/maximum inventory level   2/4
    on hand   3   reorder quantity _____

6. Tylenol #3 1000s
    minimum/maximum inventory level   1/2
    on hand   1   reorder quantity _____

7. Lipitor 10 mg
   minimum/maximum inventory level   3/10
   on hand   2   reorder quantity _____

8. Synthroid 0.05 mg
   minimum/maximum inventory level   2/4
   on hand   1   reorder quantity _____

9. Norvasc 5 mg
   minimum/maximum inventory level   3/7
   on hand   2   reorder quantity _____

10. Zoloft 50 mg
    minimum/maximum inventory level   3/5
    on hand   1   reorder quantity _____

11. Zithromax Z-Pak
    minimum/maximum inventory level   6/12
    on hand   5   reorder quantity _____

12. Toprol XL 50 mg
    minimum/maximum inventory level   1/2
    on hand   2   reorder quantity _____

13. Zocor 10 mg
    minimum/maximum inventory level   2/5
    on hand   2   reorder quantity _____

14. Prevacid 30 mg
    minimum/maximum inventory level   3/7
    on hand   3   reorder quantity _____

15. Premarin Tabs 0.625 mg
     minimum/maximum inventory level   1/2
     on hand   2   reorder quantity _____

16. Ambien 5 mg
     minimum/maximum inventory level   1/2
     on hand   2   reorder quantity _____

17. Levoxyl 0.05 mg
     minimum/maximum inventory level   2/4
     on hand   4   reorder quantity _____

18. Allegra 60 mg
     minimum/maximum inventory level   3/5
     on hand   3   reorder quantity _____

19. Celebrex 200 mg
     minimum/maximum inventory level   2/4
     on hand   3   reorder quantity _____

20. Nexium 40 mg
     minimum/maximum inventory level   3/10
     on hand   6   reorder quantity _____

21. Zyrtec 10 mg
     minimum/maximum inventory level   2/3
     on hand   3   reorder quantity _____

22. Singulair 10 mg
     minimum/maximum inventory level   3/5
     on hand   4   reorder quantity _____

23. Ultrom 50 mg
    minimum/maximum inventory level   2/5
    on hand   3   reorder quantity _____

24. Fosamax 10 mg
    minimum/maximum inventory level   2/4
    on hand   3   reorder quantity _____

25. Effexor XR 75 mg
    minimum/maximum inventory level   3/7
    on hand   5   reorder quantity _____

26. Neurontin 400 mg
    minimum/maximum inventory level   1/3
    on hand   2   reorder quantity _____

27. Celexa 20 mg
    minimum/maximum inventory level   3/6
    on hand   6   reorder quantity _____

28. Lexapro 20 mg
    minimum/maximum inventory level   2/4
    on hand   4   reorder quantity _____

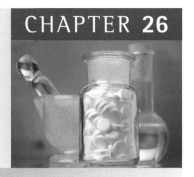

CHAPTER 26

Daily Cash Report

LEARNING OBJECTIVES

After completing this chapter, the student will be able to:

1 Describe *daily cash reports*

2 Identify the sources of payment for daily cash reports (e.g., cash, checks, bank charges)

3 Demonstrate the ability to balance a cash report

KEY TERMS

Daily cash report: format to account for the daily cash balance

Bank charges: transactions processed through credit cards

House charges: transactions processed through an in-house system for credit

Paid outs: money taken from the cash register to pay for store expenses

IN SOME RETAIL PHARMACY PRACTICES, pharmacy technicians assist the pharmacist with preparing the daily cash report for the entire store. Daily cash reports are usually prepared at the end of each business day to reflect the sales for that day. Before the cash report can be prepared, all the necessary information must be collected. An opening and closing reading is determined for each cash register. The amount of cash, checks, bank charges, other charges, and paid outs are totaled. Also, all deductions are totaled including coupons, discounts, voids, refunds, and over-rings.

℞ CAPSULE   Calculations for the total column in a cash report should always be double-checked to ensure that the vertical totals equal the horizontal totals.

Following is an example of a cash report for a drugstore/pharmacy with three cash registers.

	Reg 1	**Reg 2**	**Reg 3**	**Total**
+ Cash + Checks	1513.12	45.12	2002.02	3560.26
+ Bank Charges	120.00		350.44	470.44
+ House Charges				
+ Paid Outs				
Total	1633.12	45.12	2352.46	4030.70
+ Closing Reading	105060.56	21012.12	210121.12	336193.80
− Opening Reading	103350.54	20967.00	207768.62	332086.16
= Difference	1710.02	45.12	2352.50	4107.64
− Coupons	1.10			1.10
− Discounts	8.90			8.90
− Voids	10.00			10.00
− Refunds				
− Over-rings	56.65			56.65
Total	1633.37	45.12	2352.50	4030.99
+/−	− 0.25	0	− 0.04	− 0.29

PRACTICE PROBLEMS

STUDENT NAME _____

DATE _____   COURSE NUMBER _____

1. *Balance the following cash report:*

	Reg 1	Reg 2	Reg 3	Total
+ Cash + Checks	513.12		300.44	
+ Bank Charges	120.00			
+ House Charges			52.02	
+ Paid Outs		5.12		
Total	633.12	5.12	352.46	
+ Closing Reading	105060.56	21062.12	208121.12	
− Opening Reading	104350.54	20967.00	207768.62	
= Difference	710.02	95.12	352.50	
− Coupons				
− Discounts	8.90			
− Voids	10.00			
− Refunds				
− Over-rings	56.65			
Total	634.47	95.12	352.50	
+/−				

2. *Balance the following cash report:*

	Reg 1	**Reg 2**	**Reg 3**	**Total**
+ Cash + Checks	1145.63		4322.12	
+ Bank Charges	366.12		980.35	
+ House Charges				
+ Paid Outs				
Total				
+ Closing Reading	354632.12		17524.82	
− Opening Reading	353099.50		12222.35	
= Difference				
− Coupons	18.90			
− Discounts				
− Voids				
− Refunds				
− Over-rings				
Total				
+ / −				

3. *Balance the following cash report:*

	Reg 1	Reg 2	Reg 3	Total
+ Cash + Checks	2002.26		3601.47	
+ Bank Charges	89.12		12.99	
+ House Charges				
+ Paid Outs				
Total				
+ Closing Reading	455325.10		29159.83	
− Opening Reading	453233.55		25543.27	
= Difference				
− Coupons				
− Discounts			1.10	
− Voids				
− Refunds				
− Over-rings				
Total				
+ / −				

4. *Find the error in the following cash report, then balance the cash report:*

	Reg 1	Reg 2	Reg 3	Total
+ Cash + Checks	1513.12	45.12	2002.02	3560.26
+ Bank Charges	120.00		350.44	470.44
+ House Charges				
+ Paid Outs				
Total	1393.12	45.12	2352.46	4030.70
+ Closing Reading	105060.56	21012.12	210121.12	336193.80
− Opening Reading	103350.54	20967.00	207768.62	332086.16
= Difference	1710.02	45.12	2352.50	4107.64
− Coupons	1.10			1.10
− Discounts	8.90			8.90
− Voids	10.00			10.00
− Refunds				
− Over-rings	56.65			56.65
Total	1633.37	45.12	2352.50	4030.99
+/−	−240.25	0	−0.04	−0.29

Calculations for Institutional Pharmacy

$2\% = 2 \text{ g}/100 \text{ ml}$ $Tf = 9/5 * Tc + 32$ $2.5 \text{ gm HC}/100 \text{ gm}$

In This Section

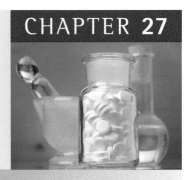

CHAPTER 27

Parenteral Doses Using Ratio and Proportion Calculations

LEARNING OBJECTIVES

After completing this chapter, the student will be able to:

1 Describe three parenteral routes of administration

2 Define *IV, IM,* and *SC*

3 Calculate parenteral doses using ratio and proportion

KEY TERMS

Parenteral medications: medications injected into the body by different routes (other than gastrointestinally)

IV: intravenous

IM: intramuscular

SC: subcutaneous

PHARMACY TECHNICIANS PREPARE parenteral medications for use in hospitals, home health care, and long term care. Parenteral medications are medications that are injected into the body by different routes such as:

■ IV (intravenous)

■ IM (intramuscular)

■ SC (subcutaneous)

Parenteral medications are available as liquids and as powders. A drug in powder form must be reconstituted before it can be injected. The strength or concentration of a medication is usually expressed as a measurement of weight (mg, g, units) in a specified volume (ml, cc). For example, 250 mg/ml or 10,000 units/2 cc.

> **℞ CAPSULE**   In pharmacy practice, milliliters (ml) and cubic centimeters (cc) are considered interchangeable.

Calculations must be made to convert the measurement of weight ordered by the physician into a volume. Different size syringes are used to measure this volume for injection, either into the patient or into a solution bag for infusion into the patient.

Ratio and Proportion Calculations

Most pharmacy calculations problems can be solved using the ratio and proportion method. A ratio expresses the relationship between two quantities. For example, 250 mg/ml means there are 250 mg of drug in each ml of solution. A proportion is an equation that states that two specific ratios are equal. The equation is written with an equals (=) sign between the two ratios. For example, 1:2 = 3:6 (1:2 is the same as 3:6).

A proportion consists of four terms. If three of the terms are known, then the fourth term (designated as X), can be calculated. When using ratio and proportion to solve a problem, each side of the equation must be set up the same—meaning that all units of measurement must be the same. (Do not mix grams and milligrams or liters and milliliters.) Always label values with the units of measurement. For example:

$$\frac{grams}{milliliters} = \frac{grams}{milliliters} \quad and \quad \frac{mg}{ml} = \frac{mg}{ml}$$

Important: Set up the proportion as ratio of drug available = ratio of drug required. That is, put the known value on the left side and unknown on the right side.

Once a proportion is set up correctly, you can solve the equation by cross multiplying.

Example

You have on hand a drug with a concentration of 250 mg/ml. How many mg are in 2 ml of the solution?

$$\frac{250 \text{ mg}}{1 \text{ ml}} = \frac{X}{2 \text{ ml}} \quad \rightarrow X \times 1 \text{ ml} = 2 \text{ ml} \times 250 \text{ mg}$$

divide each side by 1 ml and cancel out the units

$$\rightarrow \frac{X \times \cancel{1 \text{ ml}}}{\cancel{1 \text{ ml}}} = \frac{2 \cancel{\text{ ml}} \times 250 \text{ mg}}{1 \cancel{\text{ ml}}} \quad \rightarrow X = 500 \text{ mg } answer$$

Example

How many ml are needed for a 500 mg dose of a drug with a concentration of 250 mg/ml?

$$\frac{250 \text{ mg}}{1 \text{ ml}} = \frac{500 \text{ mg}}{X} \quad \rightarrow X \times 250 \text{ mg} = 1 \text{ ml} \times 500 \text{ mg}$$

$$\rightarrow \text{ divide each side by 250 mg and cancel out the units}$$

$$\rightarrow \frac{X \times \cancel{250 \text{ mg}}}{\cancel{250 \text{ mg}}} = \frac{1 \text{ ml} \times 500 \cancel{\text{ mg}}}{250 \cancel{\text{ mg}}}$$

$$\rightarrow X = 2 \text{ ml } answer$$

Example

A doctor orders a 500 mg dose of a medication. The medication is available as 1 gram per 2 ml. How many ml are needed?

Change the grams to milligrams so the units of measurement are the same:

Available 1 g / 2 ml = 1000 mg / 2 ml

Set up a ratio and proportion problem:

$$\frac{1000 \text{ mg}}{2 \text{ ml}} = \frac{500 \text{ mg}}{\text{X}} \rightarrow \text{X} \times 1000 \text{ mg} = 500 \text{ mg} \times 2 \text{ ml}$$

→ divide both sides by 1000 mg and cancel out the units

$$\rightarrow \frac{\text{X} \times \cancel{1000 \text{ mg}}}{1000 \text{ mg}} = \frac{500 \cancel{\text{ mg}} \times 2 \text{ ml}}{1000 \cancel{\text{ mg}}}$$

→ X = 1 ml *answer*

EXAMPLE

How many grams of dextrose are in 20 ml of a solution containing 50 g of dextrose in 100 ml of water?

Set up a ratio and proportion problem:

$$\frac{50 \text{ g}}{100 \text{ ml}} = \frac{\text{X}}{20 \text{ ml}} \rightarrow \text{X} \times 100 \text{ ml} = 50 \text{ g} \times 20 \text{ ml}$$

→ divide both sides by 100 ml and cancel out the units

$$\rightarrow \frac{\text{X} \times \cancel{100 \text{ ml}}}{100 \text{ ml}} = \frac{50 \text{ g} \times 20 \cancel{\text{ ml}}}{100 \cancel{\text{ ml}}}$$

→ X = 10 g *answer*

EXAMPLE

A physician orders 367.5 mg of a medication t.i.d. The drug is available as 35 mg/1 ml. What is the total in milliliters that the patient will receive in 24 hours?

Set up a ratio and proportion problem:

$$\frac{35 \text{ mg}}{1 \text{ ml}} = \frac{367.5 \text{ mg}}{\text{X}} \rightarrow \text{X} \times 35 \text{ mg} = 1 \text{ ml} \times 367.5 \text{ mg}$$

Divide both sides by 35 mg and cancel out the milligrams:

$$\rightarrow \frac{\text{X} \times \cancel{35 \text{ mg}}}{35 \text{ mg}} = \frac{1 \text{ ml} \times 367.5 \cancel{\text{ mg}}}{35 \cancel{\text{ mg}}}$$

→ X × 10.5 ml per dose

Multiple by 3 for t.i.d.:

→ 10.5 ml × 3 = 31.5 ml *answer*

Rx CAPSULE   Lumpy liquid antibiotics do not have uniform concentration of drug, and this can lead to variability in dosing.

EXAMPLE

If 0.5 ml of insulin is administered to a patient, how many units of insulin were given if the drug concentration is 1000 units/ml?

Set up a ratio and proportion problem:

$$\frac{1000 \text{ units}}{10 \text{ ml}} = \frac{X}{0.5 \text{ ml}} \quad \rightarrow X \times 10 \text{ ml} = 1000 \text{ units} \times 0.5 \text{ ml}$$

Divide both sides by 10 ml and cancel out the ml:

$$\rightarrow \frac{X \times \cancel{10 \text{ ml}}}{\cancel{10 \text{ ml}}} = \frac{1000 \text{ units} \times 0.5 \, \cancel{\text{ml}}}{10 \, \cancel{\text{ml}}}$$

$\rightarrow X = 50$ units *answer*

PRACTICE PROBLEMS

STUDENT NAME _____

DATE _____ COURSE NUMBER _____

1. A TPN requires the addition of 15 units of regular insulin U-100. A 10 ml vial of insulin contains 1000 units. How many ml of insulin should be added to the TPN? _____

0.15 ml

2. You receive an order for heparin 12,000 units in 250 ml D5W. If the strength of the heparin available is 5,000 units/ml, how many ml of heparin do you use? _____

3. Calculate the number of milliliters required to prepare the following concentrations:

   a. 25 mEq potassium chloride (stock: 2 mEq/ml KCl) _____

   b. 37.5 mg methotrexate (stock: methotrexate 50 mg/2 ml) _____

   c. 1050 mg fluorouracil (stock: fluorouracil 50 mg/ml) _____

   d. 62.5 mg doxorubicin (stock: doxorubicin 50 mg/25 ml) _____

   e. Methicillin 2.5 G (stock: methicillin 1 G/2 ml) _____

   f. Scopolamine 200 mcg (stock: scopolamine 0.4 mg/ml) _____

g. Potassium phosphate 17.6 mEq (stock: 4.4 mEq/ml potassium phosphate)   _____

h. 200,000 units penicillin (stock: penicillin 500,000 units/ml)   _____

4. If there is 20 mg of a drug in 10 ml of solution, how many liters of solution will contain 1 G of the drug?   _____

5. A vial of penicillin contains 3,000,000 units of the powdered drug. How much diluent is needed to make a solution containing 400,000 units of this drug per cc? (Assume no powder volume.)   _____

6. You have just added 0.2 ml of folic acid to an IV bag. How many mg of folic acid have you added if the stock solution contains 5 mg folic acid per ml?   _____

7. Elixir of digoxin contains 50 mcg per ml. How many mcg are in 0.3 ml of the solution?   _____

8. A physician orders 25 mg of theophylline to be given orally to a pediatric patient. If the elixir of theophylline contains 80 mg per tablespoonful, how many ml of the elixir should be administered?   _____

9. How many ml of vitamin B_{12} injection (1000 mcg/ml) must be added to an IV bag to obtain a dose of 0.5 mg of vitamin B_{12}? _____

10. A physician orders 0.4 mg of a drug. The label on the vial states that the concentration is 500 mcg per 2 ml. How many ml of the drug should be dispensed? _____

11. The doctor orders Garamycin 70 mg. A 2 ml vial contains 40 mg/ml. How many ml should be dispensed? _____

1.75

12. 7,500 units of a drug are ordered. On hand is a prefilled disposable syringe containing 10,000 units in 1 ml. How many ml should be used? _____

13. A dose of 65 units of regular insulin is to be added to a TPN bag. You are to use Humulin R (100 units/ml). How many ml would you add? _____

14. How many ml would you need for a 400 mg dose of chloramphenicol if you had a vial that contained 1 g per 10 ml? _____

15. Potassium chloride 30 mEq is to be given in 1000 ml of IV fluid. Available vials contain 40 mEq/20 ml. How many ml of the drug would you use? _____

16. How many ml of potassium chloride solution (2 mEq/ml) is required to prepare
     a liter bag of D₅W/0.2% NaCl with 25 mEq KCl?   _____

17. How many ml of aminophyllin solution (500 mg/20 ml) is needed to prepare 350 mg
     aminophyllin in 100 ml D₅W?   _____

18. Levothyroxine comes in 500 mcg vials. If the powder is diluted with 10 ml of sterile
     water, how many ml are required to provide 0.1 mg?   _____

19. You receive an order for 0.2 g of Tigan IM. You have a 5 ml vial labeled 100 mg/ml.
     How many ml are required?   _____

20. Cleocin IV comes as 600 mg/4 ml. How many ml are needed to make a piggy-back
     of 750 mg in 100 ml of 0.9% Sodium Chloride Injection?   _____

21. An injection solution is available in a 2.9 mg/5 ml concentration. A patient's required
     dose is 5.22 mg in 500 ml 0.9% sodium chloride solution. How many ml of the
     injection solution are needed?   _____

22. A drug concentration is 0.05 mg/ml in 5 ml vials. A patient requires a 0.25 mg dose. How many ml are used for this dose?   _____

23. A single IM dose of 2.4 million units of penicillin G is ordered by the physician. The concentration of the injection suspension is 600,000 units per ml in 1 ml, 2 ml, and 4 ml vials. How many ml of the suspension are required?   _____

24. Clonidine Injection is available as 10 ml vials containing 100 mcg/ml. A patient order is for 0.2 mg daily in 2 equal doses. How many ml will be needed for each dose?   _____

25. A patient is given 10.8 ml of phenytoin as a loading dose. Phenytoin is available as 50 mg per ml in 2 ml and 5 ml vials. What is the dose in mg that the patient received?   _____

26. Droperidol is available as a 2.5 mg/ml injection. A patient needs a 4 mg slow IV push. How many ml are used?   _____

27. A drug is available as 120 mcg/0.6 ml. The dose required is 100 mcg per day. How many ml will be drawn?   _____

28. A patient needs 11 million units of a drug in a single dose. The drug is available as 6 million units per ml in a 3 ml vial. How many ml will the patient receive?   _____

29. A patient requires 30 units of oxytocin by IV infusion in 1000 ml of fluid. Oxytocin is available as 10 units per ml. How many ml will the patient need?   _____

30. A patient needs a 1 G dose of streptomycin. The drug is available in a 2.5 ml vial, concentration 400 mg/ml. How many ml does the patient need?   _____

31. A 500 ml TPN needs the addition of 33 mEq of sodium chloride. The label on the vial of concentrated Sodium Chloride Injection has the following information: 30 ml single dose, 234 mg/ml, 4 mEq/ml, and 23.4%. How many ml should be added to the TPN bag?   _____

32. Digoxin Injection is available in a concentration of 0.5 mg in a 2 ml vial. The physician orders a 150 mcg dose in 150 ml of D_5W. How many ml will the patient need?   _____

33. Tobramycin Injection is available in a concentration of 80 mg per 2 ml. The patient received 1.5 ml in 100 ml of Normal Saline. What was the dose in mg that the patient received?   _____

34. Humulin R 78 units are to be added to a 1 liter TPN. The 10 ml vial of Humulin R contains 100 units/ml. How many ml are required?   _____

35. Morphine sulfate 8 mg is ordered by the physician. The label on the morphine sulfate vial reads 15 mg (1 ml fill in 2 ml size). How many ml will the patient receive?   _____

36. Atropine Sulfate Injection 0.4 mg per ml is available in the pharmacy. The doctor orders 0.8 mg. How many ml will complete this order?   _____

37. A patient requires potassium chloride 7 mEq in a 1000 ml bag of Lactated Ringers Solution. The pharmacy has on hand Potassium Chloride for Injection 40 mEq in 20 ml vials. How many ml will be needed in the IV bag?   _____

38. A patient is ordered Novolin R 54 units. The Novolin R available is 1000 units in a 10 ml vial. How many ml will the patient require?   _____

39. Aminophyllin Injection is available in a 20 ml vial containing 500 mg (25 mg/ml). The physician orders a dose of 400 mg. How many ml will be needed to fill this order?   _____

40. 500 ml of D_5W with 8,000 units of Heparin is ordered for a patient. A 5 ml vial of Heparin contains 10,000 units per ml. How many ml are needed for this patient?   _____

41. A patient order is for digoxin 0.54 mg. The injection solution is available as 250 mcg per ml. How many ml will be needed to fill the order?   _____

42. An injectable medication is available as 2 mg/ml in 1 ml and 10 ml vials.
     The patient order is for 0.5 mg in 50 ml NS IVPB tid. What is the total
     amount in ml of drug that the patient will receive per day?   _____

43. A physician order reads 3 million units of penicillin q4h. The reconstituted powder
     is available as 500,000 units/ml. What will be the total ml needed for 24 hours?   _____

44. Regular insulin is ordered for an obese patient. The drug is available in 10 ml vials
     containing 1000 units. The initial dose for the patient is 108 units in four equal doses.
     How many ml will be given for a single dose?   _____

45. Ninety-six millimols (96 mmols) of potassium phosphate is to be added to an infusion
     over 4 to 6 hours. Potassium phosphate is available as 3 mmol/ml in 5 ml, 15 ml, and
     50 ml vials. How many ml are needed for this infusion?   _____

CHAPTER 28

Powdered Drug Preparations

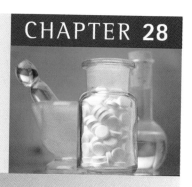

LEARNING OBJECTIVES

After completing this chapter, the student will be able to:

1 Explain why some parenteral medications are available in powder form

2 List two sources where a technician could find how much diluent is needed for reconstituting a parenteral drug

3 Calculate powder volume

4 Calculate the concentration of drug for reconstituted medications

5 Calculate the volume of reconstituted medications needed to deliver a specific dose of medication

KEY TERMS

Powdered drug preparations: drugs that have limited stability in solution and are reconstituted at the time of use from a powder form

Powder volume: the space occupied by the powder in a powdered drug preparation

Reconstitution: adding a specified amount of diluent to a powdered drug preparation before administration

SOME PARENTERAL PRODUCTS have limited stability when in solution, such as antibiotics. These drugs are supplied by manufacturers in powder form. When a powdered drug is to be administered to a patient or added to an infusion bag, it is reconstituted with a recommended diluent, usually Sterile Water for Injection. The antibiotic manufacturer's package insert includes other examples of recommended diluents.

> **Rx CAPSULE** The package insert, and sometimes the vial label, tell how much diluent to add for reconstitution. The label on the vial also indicates the amount of powdered drug contained in the vial.

The volume or space that the powdered drug occupies after it is reconstituted is called *powder volume* and is expressed in milliliters. For some drugs, the powder volume is so small that it is negligible. Other drugs have a substantial powder volume, which is always taken into consideration when reconstituting. For example, penicillin has substantial powder volume.

If the entire amount of powdered drug after reconstitution is to be used, then powder volume is not critical. However, if a partial dose is to be used, then powder volume is critical and must be calculated so that the final volume and the concentration are accurate.

Vial Size	Diluent Added	Final Volume	Powder Volume
1. 125 mg	1 ml	1 ml	None (1 ml − 1 ml)
2. 250 mg	0.9 ml	1 ml	0.1 ml (1 ml − 0.9 ml)
3. 500 mg	1.8 ml	2 ml	0.2 ml (2 ml − 1.8 ml)
4. 1 g	3.4 ml	4 ml	0.6 ml (4 ml − 3.4 ml)
5. 2 g	6.8 ml	8 ml	1.2 ml (8 ml − 6.8 ml)

EXAMPLE

The powder volume equals final volume minus the diluent added.

Increasing volumes of diluent are added to increasing vial sizes to ensure that sufficient diluent is added for dissolution. Concentrations are expressed as weight per one milliliter—for example, mg/ml, units/ml, g/ml.

EXAMPLE

What is the concentration of drug in mg/ml for each of the strengths of drug in the previous chart?

Calculate the concentration by dividing the weight of the drug in the vial by the final volume, and then reducing to milligrams in one milliliter.

1. $\dfrac{125 \text{ mg}}{1 \text{ ml}}$ − 125 mg/ml

2. $\dfrac{250 \text{ mg}}{1 \text{ ml}}$ − 250 mg/ml

3. $\dfrac{500 \text{ mg}}{2 \text{ ml}}$ reduce → $\dfrac{500 \text{ mg}/2 \text{ ml}}{2 \quad 2}$ → 250 mg/ml

4. $1 \text{ g} = 1000 \text{ mg}$ → $\dfrac{1000 \text{ mg}}{4 \text{ ml}}$ reduce → $\dfrac{1000 \text{ mg}/4 \text{ ml}}{4}$ → 250 mg/ml

5. $2 \text{ g} = 2000 \text{ mg}$ → $\dfrac{2000 \text{ mg}}{8 \text{ ml}}$ reduce → $\dfrac{2000 \text{ mg}/8 \text{ ml}}{8}$ → 250 mg/ml

EXAMPLE

You add 18 ml of Sterile Water for Injection to a vial containing 500 mg of a drug that has a powder volume of 2 ml. What is the concentration of the drug in the solution?

First, find the final volume obtained after reconstitution.

Volume of diluent   = 18 ml

Powder volume   = 2 ml
                      ————

Final volume   = 20 ml

The amount of drug in the vial = 500 mg

Calculate the concentration =

$$\frac{\text{amount of drug in vial}}{\text{Final volume}} \text{ and reduce to mg/ml}$$

$$\frac{500 \text{ mg}}{20 \text{ ml}} \text{ reduce} \rightarrow \frac{500 \text{ mg}/\cancel{20} \text{ ml}}{20 \quad \cancel{20}} \rightarrow 25 \text{ mg/ml } \textit{answer}$$

EXAMPLE

If 17 ml of Sterile Water for Injection is added to 2 g of drug and the concentration obtained is 100 mg/ml, what is the powder volume of the drug?

Set up a ratio and proportion to calculate the ml of final solution. Remember all units of measurement must be the same. 2 g = 2000 mg

$$\frac{100 \text{ mg}}{1 \text{ ml}} = \frac{2000 \text{ mg}}{X} \rightarrow \frac{X \times \cancel{100 \text{ mg}}}{\cancel{100 \text{ mg}}} = \frac{1 \text{ ml} \times 2000 \cancel{\text{mg}}}{100 \cancel{\text{mg}}}$$

$$\rightarrow X = 20 \text{ ml}$$

The final volume = 20 ml (calculated)

Diluent added   = 17 ml (given)

Powder volume   = Final volume − diluent added

                  = 20 ml − 17 ml = 3 ml *answer*

EXAMPLE

A physician orders a 750 mg dose of a medication in an IVPB. The drug is available as 15 G powder for reconstitution. The instructions state to add 26 ml of sterile water for injection to the powder to get a concentration of 500 mg/ml.

1. What is the powder volume of the drug?

   There are 15 G available. Convert this to milligrams by multiplying by 1000.

   15 × 1000 → 15,000 mg

   Set up a ratio and proportion to find the number of milliliters to give 500 mg/ml.

   $$\rightarrow \frac{500 \text{ mg}}{1 \text{ ml}} = \frac{15,000 \text{ mg}}{X} \rightarrow X \times 500 \text{ mg} = 1 \text{ ml} \times 15,000 \text{ mg}$$

   Divide both sides by 500 mg, and cancel out the mg.

   $$\rightarrow \frac{X \times \cancel{500 \text{ mg}}}{\cancel{500 \text{ mg}}} = \frac{1 \text{ ml} \times 15,000 \cancel{\text{mg}}}{500 \cancel{\text{mg}}}$$

   $$\rightarrow X = 30 \text{ ml}$$

   The instructions state to add 26 ml. The difference is the powder volume:

   $$\rightarrow 30 \text{ ml} - 26 \text{ ml} = 4 \text{ ml } \textit{answer}$$

2. How many milliliters of the reconstituted solution are needed to fill the order?

Set up a ratio and proportion using 500 mg/ml as the concentration:

➔ $\dfrac{500 \text{ mg}}{1 \text{ ml}} = \dfrac{750 \text{ mg}}{X}$ ➔ $X \times 500 \text{ mg} = 1 \text{ ml} \times 750 \text{ mg}$

Divide both sides by 500 mg, and cancel out the mg.

➔ $\dfrac{X \times \cancel{500 \text{ mg}}}{\cancel{500 \text{ mg}}} = \dfrac{1 \text{ ml} \times 750 \cancel{\text{ mg}}}{500 \cancel{\text{ mg}}}$

➔ $X = 1.5 \text{ ml}$ *answer*

PRACTICE PROBLEMS

STUDENT NAME _____

DATE _____   COURSE NUMBER _____

1. If 95 ml of Sterile Water for Injection is added to a 10 g bulk powdered drug pharmacy container, the concentration obtained is 100 mg/ml. What is the powder volume of the drug?   _____

2. Using another 10 g vial of the drug in question 1, you want a concentration of 200 mg/ml. How many ml of Sterile Water for Injection should be added? (Use the powder volume calculated in question 1.)   _____

3. The package directions for streptomycin instruct you to add 4.2 ml of Sterile Water for Injection to 1 g of dry powder to give a concentration of 200 mg/ml. What is the powder volume of the streptomycin?   _____

4. You have a vial of penicillin G potassium containing 20,000,000 units. The directions are to add 32 ml of Sterile Water for Injection to reconstitute to a concentration of 500,000 units/ml. What is the powder volume of the penicillin?   _____

5. The directions for a vial containing 500 mg of powdered Rocephin state that the addition of 1.8 ml of Sterile Water for Injection will yield a solution containing 250 mg/ml. What is the powder volume of the drug?   _____

6. If you add 8 ml of Sterile Water for Injection to a vial of 5 MU penicillin that has a powder volume of 2 ml, what is the concentration of the drug in solution?   _____

7. You add 10 ml of Sterile Water for Injection to 1 g of a drug that has a powder
    volume of 0.8 ml. What is the concentration of the drug in mg/ml in the final solution?   _____

8. If you add 27 ml of diluent to a vial containing 2.5 g of drug that has a powder
    volume of 3 ml, what will be the concentration of the drug after reconstitution?   _____

9. To prepare 3 G of Unasyn, the package insert states to add 6.4 ml of diluent.
    The concentration obtained is 375 mg/ml. What is the powder volume of the Unasyn?   _____

10. The directions for reconstitution for a 2 G vial of Claforan state to add 10 ml of
    Sterile Water for Injection to obtain a concentration of 180 mg/ml. What is the
    final volume obtained after reconstitution?   _____

11. 10 ml of Sterile Water for Injection is added to a 1 G vial of Mefoxin, giving a
    10.5 ml final volume. What is the concentration of the reconstituted powdered Mefoxin?   _____

12. A 6 G pharmacy bulk package of Fortaz is reconstituted with 26 ml of Sterile Water
    for Injection. What will be the final concentration of the drug if the powder volume
    of the Fortaz is 4 ml?   _____

13. You add 23 ml of Sterile Water for Injection to a 3 G vial of antibiotic that has a
    powder volume of 3 ml. What is the concentration, in mg/ml, of the reconstituted drug?   _____

14. A 20 G vial of a powdered drug requires the addition of 36 ml of Sterile Water for Injection to give a concentration of 500 mg/ml. What is the powder volume of the drug? _____

15. Using another 20 G vial of the drug in question 14, you need a concentration of 400 mg/ml. How many ml of Sterile Water for Injection do you need to add to the vial? _____

16. After adding 20 ml of Sterile Water for Injection to a 4 G vial of powdered drug, the concentration is 325 mg/2 ml. What is the powder volume of the drug? _____

17. A 1.5 g vial of antibiotic has a powder volume of 1.4 ml. You need a concentration of 125 mg/ml. How many ml of Sterile Water for Injection will you need to add to obtain this concentration? _____

18. Calculate the concentration, in mg/ml, after reconstitution with 19 ml of Sterile Water for Injection, of a 2.75 g vial, if the drug has a powder volume of 2.2 ml. _____

19. A technician adds 64 ml of Sterile Water for Injection to a pharmacy bulk bottle of 30 G of antibiotic powder. The antibiotic has a powder volume of 6 ml. Calculate the concentration, in mg/ml, obtained after reconstitution. _____

20. If you need a concentration of 250 mg/ml and you have on hand a 5 G vial of antibiotic with a powder volume of 1.6 ml, how many ml of Sterile Water for Injection should you add? _____

21. A 2 G vial of a drug has a powder volume of 1.5 ml.

    a. How many ml of Sterile Water for Injection will you add to obtain
       a concentration of 125 mg/ml?   _____

    b. A patient dose is 325 mg. How many ml of the reconstituted solution will you use?   _____

22. An 8 G vial of a powdered drug requires the addition of 9.8 ml of Sterile Water
    for Injection to obtain a concentration of 800 mg/ml.

    a. What is the powder volume of the drug?   _____

    b. If 2.6 ml of the reconstituted solution is added to a 500 ml bag of D5W,
       what dose (in G) will the patient receive?   _____

23. A 40 G vial of an antibiotic has a powder volume of 5.2 ml. If 94.8 ml of Sterile
    Water for Injection are added to the vial, what is the concentration (mg/ml) of the
    reconstituted solution?   _____

24. A patient is ordered a 130 mg dose of a drug in 50 ml of D_5W. A vial contains
    1 G of the powdered drug. The drug has a powder volume of 0.4 ml.

    a. How many ml of Sterile Water for Injection are needed to obtain a
       concentration of 250 mg/ml?   _____

    b. How many ml will be needed to fill the patient order?   _____

25. A 2 G vial of a powdered drug is reconstituted with 100 ml of Sterile Water for
    Injection. The drug has a powder volume of 2.3 ml. What is the concentration of
    the reconstituted solution?   _____

26. 10,000,000 units of a powdered antibiotic are contained in a vial. A concentration of 500,000 units per ml is obtained when Sterile Water for Injection is added. The drug has a powder volume of 3.2 ml. How many ml of Sterile Water for Injection should be added to the vial?   _____

27. Using another vial of the antibiotic used in question 26, if 36.8 ml of Sterile Water for Injection is added to the vial what is the concentration of the reconstituted solution?   _____

28. A 1 G vial of Nafcillin is reconstituted with 3.4 ml of Sterile Water for Injection. A concentration of 250 mg/ml Nafcillin is obtained.

    a. What is the powder volume of the Nafcillin?   _____

    b. If a patient requires a 200 mg dose in 250 ml of D_5W, how many ml of the reconstituted solution are needed?   _____

29. A powdered drug is available in vials containing 35 mg of the drug. The reconstitution instructions indicate to add 6.2 ml of Sterile Water for Injection to obtain a concentration of 5 mg/ml.

    a. What is the powder volume of the drug?   _____

    b. How many ml of the reconstituted drug are needed for a 2.5 mg dose in 50 ml NS?   _____

30. 1 ml of Sterile Water for Injection is added to a 1.5 mg vial of a powdered drug with a powder volume of 0.2 ml. What is the concentration in mg/ml of the solution obtained?   _____

31. A vial contains two different drugs. Medication A: 3.5 mg and medication B: 35 mg. The two drugs together have a powder volume of 0.5 ml. What is the concentration of each medication if 3 ml of Sterile Water for Injection is added to the vial?   _____

32. What is the powder volume of 40 G of a drug if after adding 89.6 ml of Sterile Water for Injection the concentration obtained is 400 mg/ml?   _____

33. A physician has ordered a loading dose of 600 mg in 50 ml of Normal Saline. The powder volume of the drug ordered is 0.9 ml.

   a. How many ml of Sterile Water for Injection must be added to the 5 G vial of drug to obtain a concentration of 250 mg/ml?   _____

   b. How many ml of the reconstituted solution are needed for the patient's dose?   _____

34. A 9 G vial of powdered medication is reconstituted with Sterile Water for Injection to a concentration of 300 mg/ml. How many ml of SWFI should be added if the powder volume of the drug is 1.3 ml?   _____

35. What is the concentration in G/ml of 35 G of a drug with a powder volume of 4 ml if 31 ml of Sterile Water for Injection are added to the vial?   _____

36. A patient requires 250 mcg of a medication in 50 ml of D_5W. A 4 mg vial of the medication has a powder volume of 0.1 ml 3.9 ml of Sterile Water for Injection is added to the vial.

   a. What is the final concentration of the reconstituted solution?   _____

   b. How many ml does the patient need?   _____

37. A 1.5 G vial of Unasyn contains two drugs: 1 G ampicillin and 0.5 G of sulbactam. The powder volume of the Unasyn is 0.8 ml. The label instructions indicate that 3.2 ml of SWI should be used to reconstitute the drug. What is the concentration of each of the drugs?   _____

38. A drug concentration of 250 mg/ml is needed. The powdered drug is available in a 10 G vial with a powder volume of 2.4 ml. How many ml of Sterile Water for Injection should be added to the vial to obtain the needed concentration?   _____

39. A physician orders for a patient 8 MU of a drug in 100 ml of 0.9% sodium chloride solution. The drug is available as a 20 MU powder for reconstitution with Sterile Water for Injection. The instructions are to add 32 ml of SWI to obtain a concentration of 500,000 units/ml.

   a. What is the powder volume of the drug?   _____

   b. How many ml of the reconstituted solution will the patient need?   _____

40. If 7.2 ml of SWI are added to 16 G of powdered medication with a powder volume of 0.8 ml, what is the final concentration in G/ml of the reconstituted solution?   _____

41. A powdered drug is available in 50 mg vials. The label states to add 3.8 ml of water for injection to get a concentration of 12.5 mg/ml.

   a. What is the powder volume of the drug?   _____

   b. The physician orders 18.75 mg. How many ml are needed for this dose?   _____

42.   If 0.9 ml of water for injection is added to a vial containing 0.2 mg of medication
      with a powder volume of 0.1 ml, what is the final concentration in mcg /ml?   _____

43.   3 ml of an antibiotic were added to a 50 ml IVPB. Then 5 G of the medication
      (powder volume = 0.7 ml) is reconstituted with 9.3 ml of sterile water for injection.
      How many G of the medication was added to the IVPB?   _____

44.   If 20 million units of penicillin have a powder volume of 8 ml, what is the final
      concentration for the following quantities of sterile water for injection used for reconstitution?

      a. 32 ml   _____

      b. 42 ml   _____

      c. 72 ml   _____

      d. 92 ml   _____

Percentages

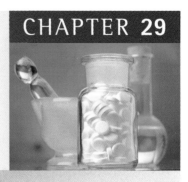

THE STRENGTHS OF MANY SOLUTIONS are expressed as a percentage. For example, 0.9% Sodium Chloride Injection; 5% Dextrose Injection. A solution is composed of two parts—the solute and the solvent:

■ The solvent is the substance (usually a liquid, but it can be a solid) in which the solute is dissolved.

■ The solute is the substance dissolved by the solvent. The percentage strength of pharmaceutical compounds is represented by a given weight, in grams, of a drug (solute) in 100 ml of solution (solvent). For example, 1 g in 100 ml = 1%; 15 g in 100 ml = 15%.

■ Dextrose Injection 5% (D_5W) contains 5 grams of dextrose per 100 ml of solution: 5 g/100 ml;

$$\frac{5 \text{ g}}{100 \text{ ml}}$$

■ Sodium Chloride Injection 0.9% (Normal Saline) contains 0.9 grams of sodium chloride per 100 ml solution: 0.9 g/100 ml;

$$\frac{0.9\ g}{100\ ml}$$

■ Concentrated Sodium Chloride Solution 23.4% contains 23.4 g of sodium chloride per 100 ml of solution: 23.4 g/100 ml;

$$\frac{23.4\ g}{100\ ml}$$

Some parenteral medications are expressed as a percentage strength. For example:

■ Magnesium Sulfate Injection 50%

■ Calcium Gluconate Injection 10%

■ Potassium Acetate Injection 19.6%

If a physician orders a dose in milligrams or grams, calculations can be made from the percentage strength concentrations.

℞ CAPSULE   Recall from Chapter 11 that percent means parts per 100 and the symbol used to express percent is %.

Example

Iodine tincture is available as a 2% solution of iodine. How many grams of iodine will be contained in 40 ml of the tincture?

$$2\% = \frac{2\ g}{100\ ml}$$

Set up a ratio and proportion using the above value.

$$\frac{2\ g}{100\ ml} = \frac{X}{40\ ml} \rightarrow \frac{X \times \cancel{100\ ml}}{\cancel{100\ ml}} = \frac{2\ g \times 40\ \cancel{ml}}{100\ \cancel{ml}} \rightarrow X = 0.8\ g\ answer$$

Example

You have 25 grams of a drug and need to compound a 30% solution. How many ml will you be able to prepare?

$$30\% = \frac{30\ g}{100\ ml}$$

Set up a ratio and proportion problem using the above value.

$$\frac{30\ g}{100\ ml} = \frac{25\ g}{X} \rightarrow \frac{X \times \cancel{30\ g}}{\cancel{30\ g}} = \frac{100\ ml \times 25\ \cancel{g}}{30\ \cancel{g}} \rightarrow X = 83.3\ ml\ answer$$

EXAMPLE

You add 80 grams of a drug to 600 ml of sterile water. What is the percentage strength of the solution prepared? Remember percentage is grams in 100 ml.

To find the percentage, find the number of grams in 100 ml.

Set up a ratio and proportion problem:

$$\frac{80 \text{ g}}{600 \text{ ml}} = \frac{X}{100 \text{ ml}} \;\rightarrow\; \frac{X \times \cancel{600 \text{ ml}}}{\cancel{600 \text{ ml}}} = \frac{80 \text{ g} \times 100 \cancel{\text{ ml}}}{600 \cancel{\text{ ml}}} \;\rightarrow\; X = 13.3 \text{ g}$$

$$\rightarrow\; 13.3\% \text{ answer}$$

There is an alternative method for solving the previous question:

$$\text{Known ratio} = \frac{80 \text{ g}}{600 \text{ ml}}$$

To find percentage multiply by 100 $\rightarrow$ $\dfrac{80 \text{ g}}{600 \text{ ml}} \times 100 = 13.3\%$ *answer*

EXAMPLE

You have an order for 2 g of calcium gluconate to add to a 1000 ml bag of 5% Dextrose Injection. The label on the calcium gluconate vial gives the concentration as 10% and 0.465 mEq/ml. How many ml will you need to use? Remember: Do not mix units.

To calculate the 2 g dose, you will use the 10% concentration, *not* the mEq/ml concentration.

Set up a ratio and proportion problem using 10% = 10 g in 100 ml.

$$\frac{10 \text{ g}}{100 \text{ ml}} = \frac{2 \text{ g}}{X} \;\rightarrow\; \frac{X \times \cancel{10 \text{ g}}}{\cancel{10 \text{ g}}} = \frac{100 \text{ ml} \times 2 \cancel{\text{ g}}}{10 \cancel{\text{ g}}} \;\rightarrow\; X = 20 \text{ ml answer}$$

EXAMPLE

The technician is to prepare 30 ml of a 20% solution using 300 mg tablets. How many tablets are needed?

The first step is to calculate the number of mg required to prepare the solution:

$$\rightarrow\; 20\% = 20 \text{ G in } 100 \text{ ml} \;\rightarrow\; \frac{20 \text{ G}}{100 \text{ ml}}$$

You need to calculate the G in 30 ml.

Set up a ratio and proportion problem:

$$\rightarrow \quad \frac{20 \text{ G}}{100 \text{ ml}} = \frac{X}{30 \text{ ml}}$$

Solve for X as previously explained in Chapter 27.

$$\rightarrow X = 6 \text{ G}$$

Convert 6 G to mg → 6 × 1000 = 6000 mg

The drug is available as 300 mg tablets.

Divide the quantity needed by the tablet strength:

$$\rightarrow \quad \frac{6000 \text{ \cancel{mg}}}{300 \text{ \cancel{mg}}}$$

$$\rightarrow 20 \text{ tablets } \textit{answer}$$

EXAMPLE

Express 0.2 mg/ml as a percentage.

Remember percentage is grams per 100 ml.

Calculate how many mg are in 100 ml.

Set up ratio and proportion:

$$\rightarrow \quad \frac{0.2 \text{ mg}}{1 \text{ ml}} = \frac{X}{100 \text{ ml}} \qquad \rightarrow \qquad X \quad = \frac{0.2 \text{ mg} \times 100 \text{ \cancel{ml}}}{1 \text{ \cancel{ml}}}$$

$$\rightarrow \qquad \qquad = 20 \text{ mg in } 100 \text{ ml}$$

Percentage is <u>grams</u> per 100 ml.

Convert 20 mg to grams.

Set up a ratio and proportion problem:

$$\rightarrow \quad \frac{1 \text{ g}}{1000 \text{ mg}} = \frac{X}{20 \text{ mg}} \qquad \rightarrow \qquad X \quad = \frac{1 \text{ G} \times 20 \text{ mg}}{1000 \text{ ml}}$$

$$\rightarrow \qquad \qquad = 0.02 \text{ G in } 100 \text{ ml}$$

$$= 0.02\% \quad \textit{answer}$$

PRACTICE PROBLEMS

STUDENT NAME_____

DATE _____ COURSE NUMBER _____

1. How many G of amino acid are in 500 ml of 8.5% solution?   _____

2. What percent strength solution would result if you mixed 3 G of NaCl in enough
    water to make 25 ml?   _____

3. A powdered drug comes in a vial containing 2.4 G. If the total volume after the
    diluent is injected is 6 ml, what is the percent strength of the solution? _____

4. A patient medication order calls for a liter bottle of acetic acid irrigation solution
    0.25%. How many mg of acetic acid are contained in each 30 ml irrigation dose? _____

5. You have dissolved 170 G of a drug in 1 liter of water. What is the percentage
    strength of the solution formed?   _____

6. You have dissolved 13.5 g of a drug in 500 ml of sterile water. What is the percentage
    strength of the solution prepared?   _____

7. On hand is a 50 ml vial of mannitol injection 25%. The order requires 3.5 G.
    How many ml should be withdrawn from the vial?   _____

8. How many mg of zinc sulfate are found in 4 oz. of a 0.02% solution?   _____

9. A solution of ampicillin contains 250 mg/ml. Calculate the percentage strength
    of the solution.   _____

10. How many grams of glucose are contained in 1500 ml of a 10% glucose solution?   _____

11. How many grams of a drug are contained in 500 ml of a 20% solution?   _____

12. How many grams of mercuric chloride are required to prepare 250 ml of a 5% solution?   _____

13. How many mg of certified red color should be used in preparing 5 liters of a
    0.01% solution?   _____

14. How many ml of a 4% stock solution of silver nitrate contain 150 mg of silver nitrate?   _____

15. How many grams of pure drug are used in preparing 250 ml of a 0.5% solution?   _____

16. How many mg of potassium chloride are in one tablespoonful of a 10% KCl solution? _____

17. How many 150 mg clindamycin capsules are needed to prepare 60 ml of a 1% clindamycin solution? _____

18. A patient is to be given 2 G of magnesium sulfate IM. The label on a 10 ml vial reads "50% solution of Mag Sulf." How many ml will you need? _____

19. You have 30 ml of 1% lidocaine on the shelf. The order calls for 40 mg. How many ml do you need to use? _____

20. You have 150 mg of cocaine to prepare a 0.4% cocaine solution. How many ml will you be able to prepare? _____

21. You need to prepare 150 G of a 2% zinc oxide ointment. How many grams of zinc oxide powder will be needed to prepare this ointment? _____

22. The pharmacy has on hand 1000 ml of an 8% sodium chloride solution. How many grams of sodium chloride are in the solution? _____

23. A technician receives an order to prepare 250 ml of a 32% sodium chloride solution. How many grams of sodium chloride crystals will the technician weigh? _____

24. A 0.3% potassium permanganate solution is ordered for a patient. The physician orders 60 ml. How many mg of potassium permanganate are needed?   _____

25. An order is received in the pharmacy for 500 G of a 27% antibiotic ointment. How many grams of the antibiotic powder will be needed to make this ointment?   _____

26. You have on hand 500 mg of a powder. How many ml of 2% solution can you prepare?   _____

27. There are 24 G of sodium chloride crystals in the pharmacy. How many liters of a 1/2% solution can the technician prepare?   _____

28. An order is sent to the pharmacy for 1.5 L of a 1/4% solution. How many grams of the powdered drug must be used?   _____

29. A technician is asked to prepare 60 ml of an 80% solution. How many grams of the solid must be weighed?   _____

30. You have in stock a 30 ml vial of 23.4% concentrated Sodium Chloride Injection.

    a. How many grams of sodium chloride are in the vial?   _____

    b. How many mg are in 1 ml?   _____

31. Calcium Gluconate is available as a 10% solution. An order is for 1.5 G of calcium gluconate. How many ml of the solution should be used?

_____

32. Hydrocortisone topical cream is available as a 0.2% concentration in 454 G. How many milligrams of hydrocortisone are in the product?

_____

33. Devonex is a topical ointment available in a 0.005% concentration. How many mg of the active ingredient are contained in 60 G?

_____

34. You have 25 mg of chloramphenicol powder in the pharmacy. How many ml of a 1% ophthalmic solution will you be able to prepare?

_____

35. You have dissolved 8.8 G of a powder in 160 ml of solvent. What is the percentage strength of the solution?

_____

36. The label on a 10 ml vial of a drug indicates a concentration of 4 mg/ml. Express this as a percentage strength.

_____

37. Co-Trimoxazole Injection contains sulfamethoxazole 80 mg and trimethoprim 16 mg per ml in 50 ml vials. What are the percentage strengths of each of the drugs?

_____

38. Co-Trimoxazole oral suspension contains sulfamethoxazole 200 mg and trimethoprim 40 mg per 5 ml. The suspension is available in 200 ml bottles. What are the percentage strengths of the two drugs?

            _____

39. You need to prepare 60 ml of a 0.025% solution. How many mg of powder will you need to dissolve?

            _____

40. A liter bag of dextrose solution contains 450 G of dextrose. What is the percentage strength of the dextrose solution?

            _____

41. The technician is asked to prepare a 15 % solution. The drug is available as 250 mg capsules. How many caps will be needed to prepare 40 ml of the solution?

            _____

42. An order reads 120 ml of 2.5 % suspension. How many 200 mg tablets will be required to fill this order?

            _____

43. A 100 ml vial of 18 % solution is available in the pharmacy. The order is for 3.6 G in a 100 ml infusion. How many ml of the solution will be used?

            _____

44. A physician orders 450 mcg of a medication. The med is available as a 0.025% solution. How many ml will be required to fill the order?

            _____

45. A medication is available as 1 G/3 ml in 20 ml vials. Express this drug concentration as a percentage strength.

            _____

CHAPTER 30

Ratio Solutions

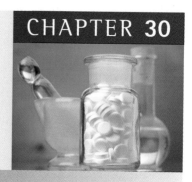

LEARNING OBJECTIVES

After completing this chapter, the student will be able to:

1 Convert ratios to fractions

2 Convert percentages to ratios

3 Convert ratios to percentages

4 Reduce ratios to lowest terms

5 Use ratio and proportion to calculate the amount of an ingredient needed to prepare a concentration of a specific ratio strength

KEY TERMS

Ratio: a comparison of one quantity to another similar quantity

Terms of the ratio: quantities compared in a ratio and separated by a colon

w/v: expression of concentration for a solid ingredient in a liquid preparation

v/v: expression of concentration for a liquid ingredient in a liquid preparation

w/w: expression of concentration for a solid ingredient in a solid preparation

THE STRENGTH of weak pharmaceutical solutions is sometimes expressed as a ratio. A ratio is a comparison of one quantity to another similar quantity. The quantities that are compared are referred to as the terms of the ratio. The terms of the ratio are written with a colon (:) between them. You will see concentrations such as 1:1000 and 1:10,000. They can also be expressed as a fraction. For example:

$$1:1000 \ \rightarrow \ \frac{1}{1000}$$

Percentages are ratios of parts per 100. For example, 5% means 5 parts per 100, or when expressed as a ratio 5:100 (said 5 in 100).

Ratio strengths are usually reduced to their lowest terms, so the first number in the ratio is a 1. To reduce a ratio where the first number is not a 1, divide both terms of the ratio by the value of the first number. For example:

5:100 can be reduced by dividing each side of the ratio by 5

$$\frac{5}{5} : \frac{100}{5} \rightarrow 1:20 \ (1 \text{ in } 20)$$

4:1000 can be reduced by dividing each side of the ratio by 4

$$4:1000 \rightarrow \frac{4}{4} : \frac{1000}{4} \rightarrow 1:250 \ (1 \text{ in } 250)$$

Ratios can be converted to percentages by changing the ratio to a fraction and multiplying by 100.

$$1:20 \quad \rightarrow \frac{1}{20} \times 100 = 5\%$$

$$1:25 \quad \rightarrow \frac{1}{25} \times 100 = 4\%$$

$$1:1000 \rightarrow \frac{1}{1000} \times 100 = 0.1\%$$

$$1:20,000 \rightarrow \frac{1}{20,000} \times 100 = 0.005\%$$

When a ratio is used to express the concentration of a pharmaceutical compound, it is interpreted as follows:

■ Solids in liquids are weight in volume solutions (w/v)

■ Liquids in liquids are volume in volume solutions (v/v)

■ Solids in solids are weight in weight compounds (w/w)

Using 1:1000 as an example:

■ a w/v solution will contain 1 g in 1000 ml of solution (1:1000 w/v)

■ a v/v solution will contain 1 ml in 1000 ml of solution (1:1000 v/v)

■ a w/w compound will contain 1 g in 1000 g of compound (1:1000 w/w)

Using 1:20 as an example:

■ a w/v solution will contain 1 g in 20 ml of solution (1:20 w/v)

■ a v/v solution will contain 1 ml in 20 ml of solution (1:20 v/v)

■ a w/w compound will contain 1 g in 20 g of compound (1:20 w/w)

EXAMPLE

How many grams of sodium bicarbonate are needed to make 200 ml of a 1:1000 w/v solution?

1:1000 w/v means 1 g in 1000 ml.

Set up a ratio and proportion problem as follows:

$$\frac{1 \text{ g}}{1000 \text{ ml}} = \frac{X}{200 \text{ ml}} \rightarrow \frac{X \times \cancel{1000 \text{ ml}}}{\cancel{1000 \text{ ml}}} = \frac{1 \text{ g} \times 200 \ \cancel{\text{ml}}}{1000 \ \cancel{\text{ml}}} \rightarrow X = 0.2 \text{ g} \ \textit{answer}$$

EXAMPLE

How many ml of boric acid solution will be required to prepare 1000 ml of a 1:20 v/v solution?

1:20 v/v means 1 ml in 20 ml

Set up a ratio and proportion problem as follows:

$$\frac{1 \text{ ml}}{20 \text{ ml}} = \frac{X}{1000 \text{ ml}} \rightarrow \frac{X \times 20 \text{ ml}}{20 \text{ ml}} = \frac{1 \text{ ml} \times 1000 \text{ ml}}{20 \text{ ml}} \rightarrow X = 50 \text{ ml } \textit{answer}$$

℞ CAPSULE Be especially careful to choose the correct strength for drugs with strengths expressed in ratios. For example, epinephrine is available in 1:1000 strength and 1:10,000 strength.

EXAMPLE

Express 1:500 as a percentage.

1:500 → 1 G in 500 ml

Remember percentage is grams in 100 ml.

Set up a ratio and proportion problem to calculate grams in 100 ml.

$$\rightarrow \frac{1 \text{ G}}{500 \text{ ml}} = \frac{X}{100 \text{ ml}} \rightarrow \frac{X = 1 \text{ G}}{500 \text{ ml}} \times 100 \text{ ml}$$

$$\rightarrow \qquad\qquad = 0.2 \text{ G in 100 ml}$$

$$\rightarrow \qquad\qquad 0.2\% \textit{ answer}$$

EXAMPLE

Express 1:2400 as a percentage.

1: 2400 → 1 G in 2400 ml.

Set up ratio and proportion as in previous example.

$$\frac{1 \text{ G}}{2400 \text{ ml}} = \frac{X}{100 \text{ ml}} \rightarrow \text{ Solve for X}$$

$$\rightarrow \quad 0.04 \text{ G in 100 ml}$$

$$\rightarrow \quad 0.04\% \textit{ answer}$$

EXAMPLE

Express 0.08% as a ratio.

0.08% is 0.08 G in 100 ml → 0.08:100

Divide both sides of the equation by 0.08 to convert the first number to 1.

$$\rightarrow \frac{0.08}{0.08} : \frac{100}{0.08}$$

$$\rightarrow \quad 1 \quad : \quad 1250 \rightarrow 1:1250 \textit{ answer}$$

PRACTICE PROBLEMS

1. You are to prepare 2 L of 1:1000 w/v Neosporin bladder irrigation. How many G of Neosporin are required?   _____

2. A 1000 ml of a 1:10 w/v sodium hypochlorite solution is ordered. How many G of sodium hypochlorite do you need to weigh?   _____

3. How many ml of a drug solution are needed to prepare 2.5 L of a 1:20 v/v solution?   _____

4. You need to prepare 750 ml of a 1:500 w/v potassium permanganate solution. How many G are needed?   _____

5. Neostigmine is available in a 1:1000 concentration in a 20 ml vial. The patient order is for 12.5 mg. How many ml are required?   _____

6. What is the percentage strength of a 1:60 solution?   _____

7. How many mg of boric acid are needed to make 150 ml of 1:400 w/v solution of boric aid?   _____

8. A prescription requires 80 mg of cocaine. On the shelf is a 1:40 w/v solution of cocaine. How many ml are needed for this prescription?   _____

9. How many G of potassium permanganate are required to prepare 500 ml of a 1:2500 w/v solution of potassium permanganate?   _____

10. You are asked to make 500 ml of a 1:10,000 w/v gentian violet solution. How many mg of the gentian violet will you need to weigh?   _____

11. Express 0.01% as a ratio.   _____

12. If 150 mg of ascorbic acid powder are mixed with 7.35 g of lactose, what is the ratio strength of ascorbic acid to lactose in the mixture?   _____

13. An order reads Adrenalin 0.4 mg SC q3h prn for asthma. Adrenalin is available in 1 ml ampoules of adrenalin 1:1000. How many ml are needed for a single dose?   _____

14. How many mg of lidocaine and epinephrine are in 20 ml of lidocaine 1% and epinephrine 1:100,000?   _____

15. Calculate the milligrams of drug needed to prepare 400 g of a 1:2500 w/w ointment.   _____

16. A technician is required to prepare 20 G of a 1:10,000 w/w ointment. How many mg of the drug are needed?

_____

17. Epinephrine is available as 1:1000 w/v solution. If the patient dose is 0.1 mg IM, how many ml are needed?

_____

18. Bupivicaine is available as a 1:400 w/v solution. The patient is given 10 ml. How many milligrams of bupivicaine did the patient receive?

_____

19. A 1:50,000 lidocaine solution is to be given to a patient. What is the concentration of the solution in mcg/ml?

_____

20. A technician is to add 1.2 mg of a drug to a 25 ml bag of 5% Dextrose Injection. On hand is a 2 ml ampoule of a 1:1000 w/v solution. How many ml should be added to the bag?

_____

21. Adrenalin Injection is available in 1 ml ampoules with a strength of 1:1000 w/v. What is the strength in mg/ml?

_____

22. Adrenalin Injection is also available as a 1:100,000 w/v strength. Express this concentration in mcg/ml.

_____

23. What is the percentage strength of a 1:100,000 w/v solution?

_____

24. A patient is to receive a medication dose of 0.5 mg in 50 ml of Normal Saline of a 1:1000 w/v solution. How many ml will be needed for this dose?   _____

25. You are to prepare 30 ml of a 1:400 w/v solution. How many mg of powdered drug will you use to make the solution?   _____

26. A technician adds 40 mg of potassium permanganate crystals to 500 ml of distilled water. What is the ratio strength (w/v) of the solution obtained?   _____

27. A patient is to receive 5 ml of a 1:2000 w/v solution. How many mg of the drug in the solution will the patient receive?   _____

28. Express 1:2000 w/v as a percentage.   _____

29. Express 0.025% as a w/v ratio.

30. A drug is available in 10 ml multiple dose vials in a concentration of 100 mcg/ml.

    a. What is the w/v ratio strength of the solution?   _____

    b. What is the percentage strength of the solution?   _____

31. A technician receives an order in the pharmacy for 750 ml of a 1:4000 w/v solution. How many mg will be needed to make this solution?   _____

32. On hand in the pharmacy is 14 G of a drug in powder form. The technician is asked to use the 14 G to make a 1:5000 w/v solution. How many liters will the technician be able to prepare?   _____

33. An order for 1 liter of a 1:4000 w/v solution is received in the pharmacy. In stock is 270 mg of the powdered drug. Will the technician be able to fill this order?   _____

34. A 2:10,000 w/v solution is available. What is the percentage strength of this solution?   _____

35. A patient requires a 100 mcg dose of a drug which is available as a 1:1000 w/v solution. How many ml of the solution will be added to a 50 ml bag of 0.9% Sodium Chloride Injection to fill the patient order?   _____

36. An order is received in the pharmacy for 50 ml of a 1:100,000 w/v solution. How many mcg are needed to fill this order?   _____

37. How many grams of a drug are needed to prepare 550 G of a 1:250 w/w ointment?   _____

38. A patient is ordered 125 mg of a drug in 500 ml of D5W solution. The concentration of the drug solution available is 1:200 w/v. How many ml of the solution will be added to the bag?   _____

39. A drug solution is labeled 1:50 w/v. What is the percentage strength of the solution?   _____

40. A technician is to prepare 150 ml of a 1:2000 w/v solution. How many mg of the drug required will be needed to prepare the solution?   _____

41. Express 0.4 % as a ratio.   _____

42. A solution is available as 0.025 % in 10 ml vials.

    a. Express the concentration as w/v ratio.   _____

    b. How many mg of the drug are in the 10 ml vial?   _____

43. Express 2:250,000 as a percentage.   _____

44. Express 40 mg/0.8 ml as

    a. a percentage.   _____

    b. a ratio.   _____

45. A patient dose is 4 ml of a 1:5000 w/v solution. How many mcg did the patient receive?   _____

CHAPTER 31

Dosage Calculations Based on Body Weight

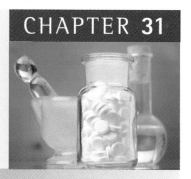

LEARNING OBJECTIVES

After completing this chapter, the student will be able to:

1 List three examples of when dosing based on body weight is important
2 Calculate medication doses based on body weight

KEY TERMS

mg/kg: milligrams of drug per kilogram of body weight

mcg/kg: micrograms of drug per kilogram of body weight

mg/lb: milligrams of drug per pound of body weight

THE BODY WEIGHT OF A PATIENT is used in calculating accurate doses of medications, especially for pediatric and geriatric patients and also for potent drugs such as chemotherapy agents. This method of calculation is considered more reliable than doses based on age. Doses are expressed as milligrams per kilogram (kg) or micrograms per kilogram or milligrams per pound of body weight: mg/kg or mcg/kg or mg/lb. Conversions from pounds to kilograms or kilograms to pounds must be made when necessary. The conversion factor is 1 kilogram (kg) = 2.2 pounds (lbs.).

> ℞ CAPSULE   Use the conversion factor 2.2 lb/kg for calculating doses based on body weight in kg.

EXAMPLE

A patient weighs 121 pounds. What is her weight in kilograms?

1 kg = 2.2 lb.

Set up a ratio and proportion problem.

$$\frac{1 \text{ kg}}{2.2 \text{ lb.}} = \frac{\text{X}}{121 \text{ lb.}} \rightarrow \frac{\text{X} \times \cancel{2.2 \text{ lb.}}}{\cancel{2.2 \text{ lb.}}} = \frac{1 \text{ kg} \times 121 \cancel{\text{ lb.}}}{2.2 \cancel{\text{ lb.}}} \rightarrow \text{X} = 55 \text{ kg } \textit{answer}$$

EXAMPLE

A patient weighs 90 kg. The dosage is based on mg/lb. body weight. What does this patient weigh in pounds?

1 kg = 2.2 lb.

Set up a ratio and proportion.

$$\frac{1\ kg}{2.2\ lb.} = \frac{90\ kg}{X} \;\rightarrow\; \frac{X \times 1\ kg}{1\ kg} = \frac{90\ kg \times 2.2\ lb.}{1\ kg} \;\rightarrow\; X = 198\ lb.\ \textit{answer}$$

EXAMPLE

A pediatric patient is ordered a 2 mg/kg single dose of a chemotherapy drug. The child weighs 44 pounds. How many mg will the child receive in the single dose?

Convert the weight from pounds to kilograms: → 1 kg = 2.2 lb.

$$\frac{1\ kg}{2.2\ lb.} = \frac{X}{44\ lb.} \;\rightarrow\; \frac{X \times 2.2\ lb.}{2.2\ lb.} = \frac{1\ kg \times 44\ lb.}{2.2\ lb.} \;\rightarrow\; X = 20\ kg$$

The dose is 2 mg/kg.

Set up a ratio and proportion.

$$\frac{2\ mg}{1\ kg} = \frac{X}{20\ kg} \;\rightarrow\; \frac{X \times 1\ kg}{1\ kg} = \frac{2\ mg \times 20\ kg}{1\ kg} \;\rightarrow\; X = 40\ mg\ \textit{answer}$$

℞ CAPSULE   Use special care when calculating doses based on body weight for children. Many serious dosing errors for pediatric patients are caused by errors in calculations.

EXAMPLE

An infant weighs 6 pounds. The dose of vancomycin to be given is 15 mg/kg/day divided into two doses. What is the dose, in mg, for one dose?

Convert 6 lb. to kg → 1 kg = 2.2 lb.

Set up a ratio and proportion:

$$\frac{1\ kg}{2.2\ lb.} = \frac{X}{6\ lb.} \;\rightarrow\; \frac{X \times 2.2\ lb.}{2.2\ lb.} = \frac{1\ kg \times 6\ lb.}{2.2\ lb.} \;\rightarrow\; X = 2.7\ kg$$

The dose is 15 mg for each kg per day.

Set up a ratio and proportion:

$$\frac{15\ mg}{1\ kg} = \frac{X}{2.7\ kg} \;\rightarrow\; \frac{X \times 1\ kg}{1\ kg} = \frac{15\ mg \times 2.7\ kg}{1\ kg}$$

→ X = 40.5 mg per day

The vancomycin is divided into two doses.

40.5 mg/2 = 20.25 mg per dose. *answer*

Doses in milliliters, for addition to infusions, can then be calculated using the concentration found on the vial label of the particular drug ordered by the physician.

EXAMPLE

A patient weighs 110 lbs. The physician orders 5 mg/kg of medication per day in 1000 ml NS. The drug is available as 50 mg/ml. How many ml will be added to the 1 L bag?

Convert 110 lbs to kg.

You may set up a ratio and proportion problem, but from previous examples, it is known that lbs divided by 2.2 = kg.

➜ $\dfrac{110 \text{ lbs}}{2.2}$ ➜ 50 kg for patient weight

The dose is 5 mg/kg ➜ 5 mg × 50 kg = 250 mg.

The medication is available as 50 mg/ml.

Set up a ratio and proportion to calculate the ml needed.

➜ $\dfrac{50 \text{ mg}}{1 \text{ ml}} = \dfrac{250 \text{ mg}}{X}$ ➜ $X = \dfrac{250 \text{ mg} \times 1 \text{ ml}}{50 \text{ mg}}$

➜ = 5 ml *answer*

PRACTICE PROBLEMS

STUDENT NAME_____

DATE _____ COURSE NUMBER _____

1. Cefuroxime is to be administered 20 mg per kg IV q4h. How many mg per dose should a child weighing 30 kg receive?   _____

2. A physician orders a medication available as 500 mg tablets for a 110-pound patient. The recommended dose for the drug is 20 mg/kg per dose. How many tablets should be given to the patient for each dose?   _____

3. The doctor orders vancomycin 10 mg/kg q12h IV for a newborn. The infant weighs 4000 g. How many mg should be given per dose?   _____

4. A physician orders cyclophosphamide to be given 5 mg/kg qid in 50 ml D_5W. The patient weighs 132 pounds. If the concentration of the drug available is 500 mg/10 ml, how many ml should be added to each bag?   _____

5. A physician requests an aminophyllin infusion. The order is for 1000 mg aminophyllin in 500 ml of D_5W. If the patient weighs 182 pounds and is to receive 0.6 mg/kg, how many ml will deliver the required dose?   _____

6. An adult intravenous dose of zidovudine is 2 mg/kg every four hours six times daily. How many mg will a 180-pound patient receive daily?   _____

7. The dose of vincristine, based on the patient's body weight, is 25 mcg/kg.
    The drug is available as 500 mcg/ml. The patient weighs 110 pounds. How
    many ml are used for a dose?   _____

8. A patient weighs 44 pounds and is receiving ampicillin at a rate of
    100 mg/kg/day. What is the total daily dose in grams?   _____

9. Calculate a single dose, in milliliters, for a 20-pound child receiving gentamicin 2 mg/kg
    of body weight IVPB q8h. Gentamicin is available in 20 mg/2 ml concentration.   _____

10. Immune globulin is available in a concentration of 6 g /100 ml. The order for a
    55-pound child is 0.2 g/kg IV. How many ml are needed for this dose?   _____

11. A 26-pound child is to receive ampicillin at a dose of 50 mg/kg/day in four equally
    divided doses. The ampicillin is available in a concentration of 125 mg/5 ml.
    How many ml are needed for one dose?   _____

12. A medication order for a patient weighing 154 pounds calls for 0.25 mg of
    amphotericin B per kg of body weight to be added to 500 ml of 5% Dextrose
    Injection. If the amphotericin B is to be obtained from a 10 ml vial containing
    50 mg, how many ml should be added to the Dextrose Injection?   _____

13. The infusion rate for theophylline for acute bronchospasm is 0.5 mg/kg/hour. How many mg of the drug will the patient receive in 24 hours, if the body weight of the patient is 100 pounds?   _____

14. A physician orders a drug 5 mg/kg three times a day for one week. What is the total daily dose, in grams, for a patient weighing 120 pounds?   _____

15. A 160-pound man is admitted to the hospital. The order states that the patient is to receive 7.5 mg/kg of acyclovir in 1000 ml of D_5W over 24 hours. The drug comes in 500 mg vials, which are diluted with 10 ml of sterile water (assume no powder volume). How many ml are to be added to the bag?   _____

16. A pediatrician has prescribed penicillin VK oral suspension for a 66-pound patient. The prescription states that the patient is to receive 50,000 units/kg/day in four equal divided doses for 10 days. On the shelf is penicillin VK 250 mg/5 ml (1500 units penicillin VK/mg). How many ml are needed for one dose?   _____

17. A five year old child weighing 45 pounds is to be given an oral dose of Tylenol Elixir. The literature states that a child of this age and weight should not exceed 71 mg/kg per day. If this daily maximum is to be divided into six doses, how much is each dose in mg? Tylenol Elixir contains 120 mg/5 ml. How many ml are needed for each of the six doses to be given?   _____

18. A 176-pound patient requires a dose of 5 mcg/kg/min of dopamine. How many mg will the patient receive in 20 minutes?   _____

19. A physician orders a bolus dose of a chemotherapy drug at a rate of 2 mg/kg. The patient weighs 200 pounds. The syringe is labeled 100 mg/5 ml. How many ml are needed for the bolus dose?   _____

20. A patient weighs 130 pounds. The physician orders gentamicin at 3 mg/kg per day in three 50 ml piggyback bags. How many mg will be added to each bag?   _____

21. Gentamycin is ordered 1.5 mg/kg/dose for a patient who weighs 135 pounds. Gentamycin is available in a 1 ml vial with a concentration of 40 mg/ml. How many ml of Gentamycin should the patient receive?   _____

22. A patient is to receive a drug IM 0.6 mg/kg every 4 hours as needed. The patient weighs 28 pounds. The drug concentration is 25 mg/ml. How many ml will the patient need per dose?   _____

23. A 64-pound child is to receive 300 mg/kg/day divided into 4 equal doses. The concentration of the drug solution available is 500 mg per ml. How many ml will the child receive for each dose?   _____

24. A physician writes an order for a 52-pound child for 400,000 units/kg/day in divided doses every 6 hours. Each dose is administered in a 50 ml bag of D_5W IVPB. The drug is available as 500,000 units per ml. How many ml will be used in each IVPB?   _____

25. A patient, weighing 80 pounds, is ordered phenobarbital 5 mg/kg at bedtime. The Phenobarbital Injection Solution is available in 1 ml vials with a concentration of 65 mg/ml. How many ml will the patient need for this dose?   _____

26. An order is received in the pharmacy for a 172-pound patient for an IV infusion of 5 mcg/kg/day in 100 ml NS. The ordered drug is available in a concentration of 300 mcg/ml in 1 ml or 1.6 ml vials. How many ml will the patient receive per day?   _____

27. Insulin is available in a concentration of 100 units/ml. A patient order reads 0.8 units/kg/day in divided doses. The patient weighs 102 pounds How many ml should the patient receive each day?   _____

28. A neonate weighs 3 1/2 pounds. She is ordered a medication dose of 20 mg/kg every 12 hours. The medication is available in a concentration of 33.3 mg/ml. How many ml will the infant require per 12 hours?   _____

29. Succinylcholine is available in a concentration of 20 mg/ml in a 10 ml vial. The order reads 40 mcg/kg every 5 to 10 minutes as a maintenance dose for the patient who weighs 190 pounds. How many ml will the patient receive for each dose?   _____

30. The drug ordered is available in the pharmacy in a concentration of 0.5 mg/ml. The physician orders a dose of 25 mcg/kg for a patient who weighs 160 pounds. How many ml will be needed to fill the order?   _____

31. Herceptin is ordered as follows:

    Dose 1:   4 mg/kg/week (1st week)
    Dose 2, 3, 4 :   2 mg/kg/week (2nd, 3rd, and 4th week)

    The patient weighs 70 kg. How many mg of Herceptin has the patient
    received after 4 weeks?

    _____

32. A physician orders a medication for a patient who weighs 130 pounds. The order
    reads 300 mg/kg in 50 ml D_5W q4h. How many grams of the medication will the
    patient receive in 24 hours?

    _____

33. A patient order is for 1.5 G/kg by slow infusion. The patient weighs 145 pounds.
    The drug concentration is 40 G/150 ml. How many ml will the patient need?

    _____

34. A patient needs 4400 units/kg/hour of a drug for a 12-hour infusion. The patient
    weighs 172 pounds. What is the total number of units the patient will receive over
    the 12-hour infusion?

    _____

35. Zinc Sulfate Injection is available in a concentration of 1 mg/ml. An order is received in
    the pharmacy for a five year old child who weighs 49 pounds. The order reads 100 mcg/kg
    per day. How many ml will the child receive in one day?

    _____

36.   A patient is to receive a course of treatment over 3 days. The patient weighs 122 pounds. The dosage is as follows:

Day 1: 10 mg/kg
5 mg/kg 6 hours later
Day 2, 3: 5 mg/kg

What is the total amount of drug in grams that the patient will need over the course of the treatment?

37.   Ceftazidime is ordered for a 52-pound patient at a dosage of 50 mg/kg/dose every 8 hours. The drug in solution is available in a concentration of 100 mg/ml. How many ml are required for each dose?

38.   The dose for a newborn is 800 mg/kg/day as a continuous infusion. The infant weighs 7.5 pounds. The drug is available as a 100 mg/ml solution. How many ml are needed for the dose?

39.   A drug is available as 39.55 mg/ml in a 10 ml vial. The patient order received in the pharmacy is for 35 mg/kg/day. The patient weighs 109 pounds. How many ml are required to fill the order?

40.   A 139-pound patient is ordered a medication dose of 125 mg/kg/24 hours. The concentration of the medication to be used is 425 mg/2 ml. How many ml are needed for the patient dose?

41. A pediatric patient order is 75 mcg/kg q12h. The patient weighs 33 lbs. The medication is available as 1 mg/ml. How many ml will be needed over 24 hours?

        _____

42. Potassium chloride is ordered 0.5 mEq/kg/hr for a patient who weighs 154 lbs. The potassium chloride label reads 2 mEq/ml. How many ml are needed for a 4-hour infusion in 1000 ml D5W?

        _____

43. A patient weighing 132 lbs is ordered theophylline 0.55 mg/kg/hr for 12 hours. What is the total amount of theophylline in mg that will be administered?

        _____

44. A neonate order is 0.03 mg/kg of a 1:10,000 solution. The patient weighs 4.4 lbs. How many ml of the solution will be needed?

        _____

45. Cimetidine is available as an injection solution with a concentration of 150 mg/ml. The patient weighs 66 lbs. The dose ordered is 20 mg/kg/day in divided doses q6h. How many ml will be needed for each dose?

        _____

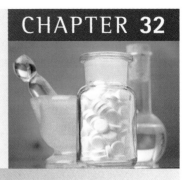

CHAPTER 32

Dosage Calculations Based on Body Surface Area

LEARNING OBJECTIVES

After completing this chapter, the student will be able to:

1 Identify which types of drugs are dosed according to body surface area

2 Use a nomogram to calculate body surface area

3 Perform dosing calculations for drugs based on body surface area

KEY TERMS

BSA: body surface area (expressed in m²)

Nomogram: chart used to calculate body surface area as a function of height and weight

BODY SURFACE AREA (BSA) is used to accurately calculate doses for patients receiving chemotherapy agents. BSA is expressed as square meters (m²). Body surface area is calculated using patient body weight and height, and can be determined by referring to a standard nomogram.

A nomogram has three columns:

■ Height (expressed in centimeters and in inches)

■ Body surface area (expressed in square meters)

■ Weight (expressed in kilograms and in pounds)

The height and weight of the patient are found on the nomogram and then a straight line is drawn connecting the two values. The BSA for that patient is found where the line intersects the BSA column. Many manufacturers of chemotherapy drugs supply BSA calculators with sliding scales. The principle of finding the BSA is similar to the nomogram.

> **℞ CAPSULE** Use a straight edge (such as a ruler) when using a nomogram to calculate BSA. Simply align the straight edge so it intersects at the height and weight and determine the BSA by reading the value at the intersection in the BSA scale.

EXAMPLE

A physician orders a chemotherapy drug in a dose of 5 mg/m². If the patient has a BSA of 2.1 m², what will be the dose in mg?

Set up a ratio and proportion:

$$\frac{5 \text{ mg}}{1 \text{ m}^2} = \frac{X}{2.1 \text{ m}^2} \;\rightarrow\; \frac{X \times 1 \text{ m}^2}{1 \text{ m}^2} = \frac{5 \text{ mg} \times 2.1 \text{ m}^2}{1 \text{ m}^2} \;\rightarrow\; X = 10.5 \text{ mg} \;\; answer$$

EXAMPLE

The physician orders a drug for a child with a BSA of 0.95 m². The drug dose is 750 mcg/m². What will be the dose in milligrams for this child?

Set up a ratio and proportion:

$$\frac{750 \text{ mcg}}{1 \text{ m}^2} = \frac{X}{0.95 \text{ m}^2} \;\rightarrow\; \frac{X \times 1 \text{ m}^2}{1 \text{ m}^2} = \frac{750 \text{ mcg} \times 0.95 \text{ m}^2}{1 \text{ m}^2} \;\rightarrow\; X = 712.5 \text{ mcg}$$

The dose is in mg   1 mg = 1000 mcg

To find the number of milligrams, divide the micrograms by 1000.

$$\frac{712.5 \text{ mcg}}{1000} = 0.713 \text{ mg } answer$$

EXAMPLE

Using the nomogram: A patient's weight is 80 kg and height is 6'6". The physician orders his chemotherapy treatment as 6.5 mg/m² once daily for five days. How many mg of drug will the patient receive in one day?

From the nomogram BSA = 2.30 m²

Set up a ratio and proportion:

$$\frac{6.5 \text{ mg}}{1 \text{ m}^2} = \frac{X}{2.30 \text{ m}^2} \;\rightarrow\; \frac{X \times 1 \text{ m}^2}{1 \text{ m}^2} = \frac{6.5 \text{ mg} \times 2.30 \text{ m}^2}{1 \text{ m}^2} \;\rightarrow\; X = 14.95 \text{ mg} \;\; answer$$

EXAMPLE

Using the nomogram provided, find the BSA for the following patient.

                    Patient 1   →   weight 50 kg; height 55 inches

Using a straight edge (a ruler is good), find the patient weight and height and place the ruler on each. Where the ruler intersects with the BSA (the middle line) is the BSA for the patient.

                                     →   BSA = 1.40 m²

                    Patient 2   →   weight 84 lb; height 119 cm;   BSA = 1.10 m²

                    Patient 3   →   weight 60 kg; height 150 cm;   BSA = 1.59 m²

Practice using the nomogram accurately.

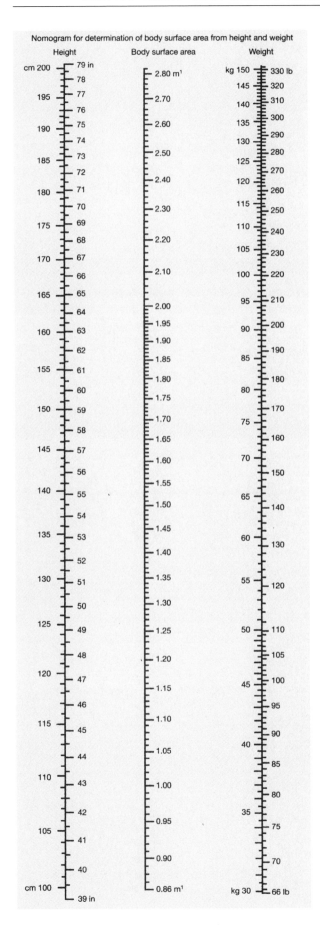

Nomogram for determination of body surface area from height and weight

Students and teachers should use this nomogram for calculations in this textbook. To use another nomogram may give different answers.

From the formula of Du Bois and Du Bois, *Arch. inture. Med.*, 17, 863 (1916): $S = W^{8.466} \times H^{8.766} \times 71.84$, or $\log S = \log W \times 0.425 + \log H \times 0.725 + 1.8564$ (S = body surface in cm², W = weight in kg, H = height in cm). From *Scientific Tables*, 7th ed. Basel, J. R. Geighy, p. 537.

PRACTICE PROBLEMS

STUDENT NAME _____

DATE _____   COURSE NUMBER _____

1. A physician orders a bolus dose of doxorubicin for a patient with a BSA of 0.96 m². The drug dose is 75 mg/m². What is the bolus dose in mg?   _____

2. A patient weighs 98 pounds and is 5'1" tall. Using the nomogram, find the patient's BSA. The dose of vincristine ordered by the physician is 10 mg/m² per day. What will be the dose in mg? _____

3. A patient with a BSA of 1.95 m² is ordered a dose of doxorubicin of 40 mg/m² two times daily. What will be the daily dose, in mg, for this patient?   _____

4. Using the nomogram, find the BSA for the following patient: Weight is 64 kg, height is 5'6". The physician orders a dose of vinblastine of 1.6 mg/m² daily for four days. Calculate the number of milligrams received by the patient over the four days.   _____

5. A patient's weight is 70 kg and height is 155 centimeters. Calculate the dose of fluorouracil, in mg, for the patient if the oncologist orders 400 mg/m² daily.   _____

6. A patient has a BSA of 1.54 m². The physician orders a daily dose of 900 mg/m² of methotrexate for this patient. What is the daily dose, in ml, if the concentration of methotrexate available is 25 mg/ml?   _____

7. A physician order is for Adriamycin 25 mg/m² daily for four days. The patient has a 2.5 m² BSA. What is the total amount, in mg, that the patient will receive over the four days? _____

8. A patient with 1.8 m² BSA is to receive mesna 4500 mg/m² IV in 1000 ml D₅W over 18 hours on day one of treatment. Mesna is available as 1000 mg/ml vials. Calculate how many ml are required for the IV bag. _____

9. The physician for a patient, BSA 1.9 m², orders cisplatin 15 mg/m² continuous infusion. Cisplatin is available in 50 ml vials with a concentration of 1 mg/ml. How many ml will be required for this order? _____

10. Taxotere is ordered 55 mg per m² over one hour. The patient has a BSA of 1.93 m². Taxotere is available in a concentration of 20 mg/ml. Calculate how many ml are needed for this patient's dose. _____

11. A patient weighs 184 pounds and is 72 inches in height. The physician orders doxorubicin 25 mg/m² IV push. The doxorubicin is supplied as 50 mg vials reconstituted to 4 mg/ml. How many ml will this patient need for his IV push? _____

12. A patient with a BSA of 1.52 m² is ordered leukovorin 100 mg/m² IV in 100 ml 0.9% sodium chloride solution over one hour. Leukovorin is supplied as 200 mg dry powder that is reconstituted to 10 mg/ml. Calculate how many ml are to be added to the IV bag. _____

13. 5FU 400 mg/m^2 as IV push is ordered for a patient—whose height is 60.5 inches and weight is 123.4 pounds. 5FU is available as 50 mg/ml in 10 ml vials. How many ml will the patient require?   _____

14. Topetecan 1 mg/m^2 IV over 30 minutes in 50 ml of Normal Saline is ordered for a patient with a BSA of 2.00 m^2. Topetecan is supplied as 4 mg/vial reconstituted to 1 mg/ml. How many ml will be added to the IV bag?   _____

15. A patient with a BSA 1.8 m^2 is to receive Cytoxan 4500 mg/m^2 IV in 1000 ml of 0.9% Sodium Chloride Injection over 12 hours. Cytoxan is supplied as 2 g vials 50 mg/ml after reconstitution. How many ml should the technician add to the IV bag?   _____

16. A patient with a BSA of 1.52 m^2 is to receive etoposide 2000 mg/m^2 via a syringe pump over two hours. Etoposide is supplied as 525 mg/25 ml vials. How many ml will be needed for this patient?   _____

17. Bleomycin 10 units/m^2 IV push is ordered for a patient with a BSA 2.05 m^2. Bleomycin is available as 15 units/ml. Calculate how many ml are needed for this patient's dose.   _____

18. A patient, whose weight is 80.5 kg and height is 63 inches, is to receive dacarbazine 375 mg/m^2 in 250 ml 5% Dextrose Injection over 30 to 60 minutes. Dacarbazine is available as 200 mg/vial reconstituted to 10 mg/ml. How many ml will be needed to add to the IV bag?   _____

19. Paclitaxel 45 mg/m^2 in 500 ml Normal Saline is to be given to a patient with BSA 2.1 m^2. Paclitaxel is supplied as 6 mg/ml. How many ml should the technician add to the IV bag?   _____

20. A physician orders carboplatin, 360 mg/m^2 in 250 ml Normal Saline infused over one hour. The patient has a BSA of 2.6 m^2. How many ml must the technician add to the IV bag? Carboplatin is available after reconstitution in a concentration of 10 mg/ml.   _____

21. A physician orders a 375 mg/m^2 dose of Rituxan in 500 ml NS for a patient with a BSA of 1.24 m^2. Rituxan is available in 10 ml vials in a concentration of 10 mg/ml. How many ml will be added to the IV bag?   _____

22. Cyclophosphamide, after reconstitution, has a concentration of 20 mg/ml. The patient, who weighs 67 kg and is 155 cm tall, is ordered cyclophosphamide 600 mg/m^2 in 250 ml NS. How many ml will be added to the bag?   _____

23. Doxorubicin, after reconstitution, is available as a 2 mg/ml solution. The physician orders a syringe for IV push at a dose of 35 mg/m^2. The patient has a BSA of 1.2 m^2. How many ml are drawn into the syringe?   _____

24. A patient is to receive Taxol 175 mg/m^2. She weighs 90 pounds and is 5'2" tall. The Taxol is available, after reconstitution, in a concentration of 6 mg/ml. How many ml will be added to a 500 ml bag of NS for IV infusion?   _____

25. An order is received in the pharmacy for 5-FU IV for a patient with a BSA of 1.6 m². The 5-FU solution is available in a 50 mg/ml concentration. The dosage schedule is as follows:

    Initial dose: 400 mg/m² for 5 days IV push

    How many grams of 5-FU has the patient received for the initial dose?   _____

26. 50 mg of a powdered drug is reconstituted with 10 ml of Sterile Water for Injection (assume no powder volume). A patient is ordered an 85 mg/m² dose of the drug in 250 ml D₅W. The patient's BSA is 0.82 m². How many ml of the reconstituted drug will be added to the IV bag?   _____

27. A patient weighs 180 pounds and is 6'2" tall. The dose of a drug ordered by his physician is 1.3 mg/m² IV push twice weekly for two weeks. The drug is available in a concentration of 1 mg/ml. How many ml of the ordered drug will the patient receive for each dose?   _____

28. A patient, weight 125 pounds, height 5'6", is to receive the following chemotherapy regime: 800 mcg/m² twice weekly for 2 weeks. The chemo drug when reconstituted has a concentration of 1 mg/ml. How many ml of the drug will the patient receive for the complete regime?   _____

29. The initial loading dose of a chemo drug is 400 mg/m² infused over 120 minutes and the maintenance dose is 250 mg/m² infused over 60 minutes. The drug is available as 12 mg/ml. The patient, BSA 1.2 m², received a 25 ml dose. Is this an initial or maintenance dose?   _____

30. A physician orders bleomycin in a dose of 20 units/m² twice weekly. The reconstituted bleomycin has a concentration of 30 units/5 ml. The patient has a BSA of 2.5 m². How many ml will the patient need for a single dose?

_____

31. An order is received in the pharmacy for methotrexate 40 mg/m². Methotrexate is available in a concentration of 2.5 mg/ml. How many ml are needed for the dose for the patient (weight 80 kg, height 160 cm)?

_____

32. A physician orders mesna 1.33 G/m²/day. The pharmacy has on hand mesna 100 mg/ml. The patient has a BSA of 0.8 m². How many ml will the patient receive each day?

_____

33. A 155-pound patient (height 5'9") is ordered interferon Alfa-2b IM 2 million units/m² 3 times a week. The drug is available 10 MU in 1 ml. How many ml will the patient need per week?

_____

34. In the pharmacy, idarubicin is available as a 1 mg/ml solution for IV use. The patient, with a BSA of 1.5 m² is ordered 12 mg/m²/day for 3 days by slow IV. How many ml will be administered for the total treatment?

_____

35. 20 ml Sterile Water for Injection is added to a 1 G vial of powdered ifosfamide (assume no powder volume). The order for the patient is 700 mg/m² IV push. How many ml of the reconstituted ifosfamide will be drawn into the syringe? The patient has a BSA of 1.1 m².

_____

36. The patient is to receive a rapid bolus dose of Alkeran within the hour. The order is for 16 mg/m². Alkeran is reconstituted to 5 mg/ml. The patient has a BSA of 1.92 m². How many ml of the reconstituted solution will the patient need? _____

37. Robaxin Injection is available in a 10 ml vial with a concentration of 100 mg/ml. An order is received in the pharmacy for Robaxin Injection 500 mg/m²/dose that may be repeated in 6 hours. The patient weighs 68 pounds and is 4'10" tall. How many ml will the patient need for one dose? _____

38. A 1 G vial of methotrexate when reconstituted with Normal Saline has a concentration of 50 mg/ml. A patient with a BSA of 1.39 m² is ordered 6 G/m² by IV infusion every week. How many ml of the reconstituted solution will the patient receive? _____

39. A chemo drug is available in the pharmacy as 50 mg capsules. A patient with a BSA of 1.66 m² is ordered 60 mg/m²/day for 14 days. How many capsules will the patient require for this course of treatment? _____

40. Leukine is to be administered by IV at 250 mcg/m²/day for 21 days. The standard diluted dose in use is 250 mcg/25 ml NS. How many ml will a patient with a BSA of 2.1 m² require each day? _____

41. Cytarabine is available as a 20 mg/ml injection. A patient with a BSA of 1.4 m^2 is to receive 75 mg/m^2/day for 10 days. How many ml will be administered IV each day?   _____

42. A high dose 3.38 G/m^2 of dacarbazine is ordered for a patient with a BSA of 1.5 m^2. The medication is available after reconstitution as 20 mg/ml. How many ml will be required for the IV infusion?   _____

43. A chemo drug is available as 5 mg/ml. A patient with a BSA of 0.99 m^2 is ordered 25 mg/m^2. How many ml are needed?   _____

44. A child with a BSA of 0.97 m^2 is ordered a one-time dose of 12 mg/m^2. The antineoplastic is available as 1 mg/ml in 10-ml vials. How many ml are required for the one dose?   _____

45. A patient with a BSA of 2.1 m^2 is to receive 7.5 mg/m^2/week of methotrexate. MTX is available as 25 mg/ml. How many ml are needed for the weekly dose?   _____

Infusion Rates and Drip Rates

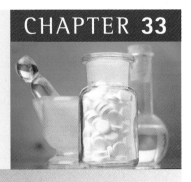

LEARNING OBJECTIVES

After completing this chapter, the student will be able to:

1 Calculate the rate of infusion if the volume of infusion and the time of the infusion are known

2 Calculate the rate of flow for an IV in drops/min if the calibration of the IV set is known along with the volume of the infusion and the time of the infusion

3 Calculate the rate of flow for an IV in ml/hour if the volume of the infusion and the time of the infusion is known

KEY TERMS

Infusion rate: the volume of solution or drug to be administered in a set amount of time for an intravenous preparation

ml/min: milliliters of IV solution administered per minute

ml/hr: milliliters of IV solution administered per hour

mg/min: milligrams of drug administered per minute

drops/min: drops of IV solution administered per minute

IV set: tubing and equipment for delivering IVs

Calibrated: the number of drops per ml for a given IV set

PHYSICIANS WRITE ORDERS for the rate at which an IV is infused into a patient. Infusion rates can be expressed as number of milliliters per minute, milliliters per hour, amount of drug per hour, and often as the length of time for a volume to be infused. For example:

■ Infuse at 125 ml/hr

■ Infuse 1000 ml over 8 hours

■ Infuse 10 mg per minute

If the volume of the infusion and the time of the infusion are known, then the rate of infusion can be calculated from the following formula:

$$\frac{\text{Volume}}{\text{Time}} = \text{Rate}$$

EXAMPLE

Infuse 1000 ml over 8 hours. What is the rate of infusion in ml/hr?

$$\frac{1000 \text{ ml}}{8 \text{ hr}} = \text{Rate} \rightarrow 125 \text{ ml/hr}$$

The time of an infusion can be calculated using the same formula. For example, if the rate of infusion is 100 ml/hr and the volume of the infusion is 1000 ml, how long will this bag last?

$$\frac{1000 \text{ ml}}{\text{Time}} = 100 \text{ ml/hr} \rightarrow \text{Time} = \frac{1000 \text{ ml}}{100 \text{ ml/hr}} \rightarrow 10 \text{ hours}$$

Similarly, the volume of an infusion can be calculated using the same formula.

Infusions that are administered to a patient by gravity flow are infused through IV sets that are calibrated in drops per milliliter. The rate of infusion is expressed as drops per minute.

Conversions are made to a flow rate of drops per minute from the infusion rate ordered by physicians.

To convert a flow rate in ml/hr to drops/min, two steps are involved.

> ℞ CAPSULE   To convert a flow rate in ml/hr to drops/per min two conversion factors are needed. The first conversion factor is 60 min/hr and the second conversion factor is to determine drops/ml. The number of drops/ml is determined by the size of the tubing and the nature of the administration set.

EXAMPLE

The flow rate of an IV infusion ordered by a physician is 125 ml/hr. The IV set to be used for the infusion is calibrated at 15 drops/ml. Calculate the rate of flow in drops/min.

Convert the flow rate from ml/hr to ml/min. 1 hour = 60 minutes

Set up a ratio and proportion.

$$\frac{125 \text{ ml}}{60 \text{ mins}} = \frac{X}{1 \text{ min}} \rightarrow \frac{X \times 60 \text{ min}}{60 \text{ min}} = \frac{125 \text{ ml} \times 1 \text{ min}}{60 \text{ min}}$$

$$\rightarrow X = 2.08 \rightarrow 2.1 \text{ ml/min}$$

Calculate the drops for 2.1 ml/min using the calibration of the IV set → 15 drops/ml.

Set up a ratio and proportion.

$$\frac{15 \text{ drops}}{1 \text{ ml}} = \frac{X}{2.1 \text{ ml}} \rightarrow \frac{X \times 1 \text{ ml}}{1 \text{ ml}} = \frac{15 \text{ drops} \times 2.1 \text{ ml}}{1 \text{ ml}}$$

$$\rightarrow X = 31.5 \rightarrow 32 \text{ drops/min } \textit{answer}$$

All conversions from ml/hr to drops/min can be calculated using this two-step method.

EXAMPLE

A physician orders 12,500 units of heparin in a 1000 ml bag of 5% Dextrose Injection for a patient. The rate of infusion is 500 units over one hour. What will be the rate of infusion in ml/hour?

Calculate the volume, in milliliters, that will contain 500 units.

Set up a ratio and proportion problem.

$$\frac{12,500 \text{ units}}{1000 \text{ ml}} = \frac{500 \text{ units}}{X}$$

Cross-multiply and divide both sides by 12,500 units.

$$\rightarrow \frac{X \times \cancel{12,500 \text{ units}}}{\cancel{12,500 \text{ units}}} = \frac{1000 \text{ ml} \times 500 \cancel{\text{units}}}{12,500 \cancel{\text{units}}}$$

$\rightarrow$ X = 40 ml/hr *answer*

EXAMPLE:

A 1-liter bag of D_5W is to be run at 100 ml/hr. The bag is started at 8:00 am. What time will the bag finish?

1 liter = 1000 ml

1000 ml at 100 ml/hr

Set up a ratio and proportion to calculate how long the bag will take to finish.

$$\frac{100 \text{ ml}}{1 \text{ hr}} = \frac{1000 \text{ ml}}{X} \quad \rightarrow \quad X = \frac{1000 \cancel{\text{ml}} \times 1 \text{ hr}}{100 \cancel{\text{ml}}}$$

$$\rightarrow = 10 \text{ hr}$$

The bag is started at 8:00 am and will finish 10 hours later.

$\rightarrow$ 6:00 pm *answer*

PRACTICE PROBLEMS

STUDENT NAME _____

DATE _____ COURSE NUMBER _____

1. If a 1 liter bag of D_5W is run through an IV into a patient's arm over eight hours, what is the rate of infusion in ml/hr?   _____

2. If a 500 ml bag of 0.9% Sodium Chloride Injection is run over eight hours, what is the rate of infusion?   _____

3. If a 1000 ml bag of Normal Saline is run at 100 ml/hr, how long will the bag last?   _____

4. A sterile solution request form is received for a large volume parenteral. The infusion rate is 125 ml/hr. The nurse requests enough 1 liter bags for the next 24 hours. How many bags do you make?   _____

5. If the infusion rate for an IV is 80 ml/hr and it is run for four and a half-hours, how many ml has the patient received?   _____

6. If 1 liter of D_5W is started on a patient at 1400 hours on Tuesday, at what time and day will the next liter be required if the rate is:

    a. 125 ml/hr   next bag needed at _____ on _____ day

    b. 80 ml/hr   next bag needed at _____ on _____ day

    c. 200 ml/hr   next bag needed at _____ on _____ day

    d. 50 cc/hr   next bag needed at _____ on _____ day

7. Potassium chloride 30 mEq is to be given in 1 liter of IV fluid. The infusion
    rate is 125 ml/hr. How many mEq/hr are being infused?   _____

8. A 50 ml IVPB bag of ampicillin 500 mg in Normal Saline is to be run in over
    20 minutes. What is the infusion rate in ml/hr?   _____

9. An order is for heparin IV to infuse at 1000 units per hour. What will be the
    flow rate in ml/hr for a 500 ml bag of D_5W with 25,000 units of heparin?   _____

10. A patient is on a heparin drip, 12,500 units in 250 ml of 0.45% Sodium Chloride Injection.
    He is to receive 1500 units per hour. At what rate (ml/hr) should the drug be infused?   _____

11. How many drops per minute will a patient receive if an IV of 1000 ml of 5%
    Dextrose Injection is run in over eight hours? The drip factor is 15 drops/ml. _____

12. One hundred micrograms of a drug, dissolved in 240 ml of solution, is to be infused at a rate of 75 mcg/hr. If 1 ml = 15 drops, what should the rate of administration be in drops/min? _____

13. Calculate the infusion rate in ml/hr for a drip, concentration 5 gm/500 ml. The rate is 25 mcg/kg/min. The patient weighs 112 kg. _____

14. What is the flow rate, in drops/min, for a TPN compounded with 500 ml of $D_{10}W$ and 500 ml 7% Travasol run in over 24 hours? The IV administration set is calibrated to deliver 10 drops/ml. _____

15. The physician orders 3000 ml of D_5W IV over a 24-hour period. If the IV set is calibrated to deliver 15 drops per ml, how many drops must be administered per minute? _____

16. How long will it take to complete an IV infusion of 1.5 L of 0.9% Sodium Chloride Injection being administered at 45 drops/minute? The IV set is calibrated to deliver 15 drops per ml. _____

17. Ampicillin 500 mg in 50 ml IVPB is to be administered over a period of 15 minutes. The drop factor for the IV administration set is 10 drops/ml. Calculate the rate of flow in drops per minute.   _____

18. The drop factor for an IV line is set at 30 drops/min. Calculate the rate of infusion in ml/hr. The drop factor is 15 drops/ml.   _____

19. You have a 500 ml bottle of an 8% drug. The rate of infusion is 5 g/hr. What is the rate of infusion in ml/hr and how long will the bottle last?   _____

20. What volume of fluid will a patient receive if a large volume parenteral bag is running at 50 ml/hr and is begun at 0800 and discontinued at 1400?   _____

21. A physician orders an IV to be infused at 30 mg/minute for 24 hours. What is the total gram dose for this patient?   _____

22. A patient is to receive 2 G of an antibiotic in 250 ml of D$_5$W/NS over 1 hour. The rate of infusion is 30 mg/minute. How long will it take for the patient to receive the infusion?   _____

23. The rate of infusion of a drug is 45 ml/hr as ordered by the physician. A bag of 1000 ml of D$_5$W is hung on day 1 at 0400 hours. What time will the next 1000 ml bag be needed?   _____

24. A 50 ml IVPB bag contains 500,000 units of penicillin G. The rate of infusion ordered by the physician is 120 ml/hr. How long will the IVPB take to infuse?   _____

25. An IV is running at 50 ml/hr. The 500 ml bag contains 180 mEq of potassium chloride. How many mEq of potassium chloride is the patient receiving per hour?   _____

26. A physician orders a drug to be infused at 10 mcg/kg/min. The patient weighs 70 kg. The total dose the patient is to receive is 21 mg. How long must the IV continue for the patient to receive this dose?   _____

27. A patient order is for 1000 ml to be infused over 75 minutes. What is the rate of
     infusion in ml/hr?   _____

28. The infusion rate for 50 ml of D_5W containing 3.5 G of an antibiotic is 200 ml/hr.
     What is the infusion rate in drops/min if the IV set is calibrated at 10 drops/ml?   _____

29. A 500 ml IV bag of Lactated Ringers is to be infused at 100 ml/hr. How many 500 ml
     bags will be needed for 24 hours?   _____

30. A 250 ml bag of D_5W is to be infused at 40 drops/min. The IV set drop factor is
     60 drops/ml. The IV is started at 6 a.m. When will the next bag be needed?   _____

31. The physician orders a 500 mg loading dose of a drug to be administered over
     20 minutes by IV infusion. A 50 ml IVPB containing the 500 mg is supplied.
     At what rate in ml/hr should the IVPB be infused?   _____

32. An order is received to infuse 750 ml of IV fluid every 6 hours. At what rate
     should the IV pump be set for (in ml/hr)?   _____

33. A patient is receiving 250 ml of D$_5$W infusing at 33 gtt/min. The IV tubing is calibrated for 10 gtt/ml. What is the infusion time for the bag? _____

34. An MD orders a continuous infusion at a rate of 3 ml/min. The 1000 ml IV bag contains a 2 G dose of the medication ordered. How many mg of the drug will the patient receive in 20 minutes? _____

35. 37 units of Regular Insulin is to be administered over 1 hour as a continuous infusion. The insulin is added to a 250 ml bag of 0.9% Sodium Chloride Solution. What infusion rate (gtt/min) should be used if the IV set is calibrated for 10 drops/ml? _____

36. A medication is ordered by the physician 2 G in 250 ml NS to be administered by continuous IV around the clock for 24 hours. The rate of infusion is 100 ml/hr. If the first bag is started at 0800, how many bags in total will be needed? _____

37. With reference to question 36, give the times (in military time) that each bag will be started. _____

38. A continuous infusion is to be administered at a rate of 2 mg/min. 200 mg of the drug is added to 250 ml of Ringers Solution. What is the rate of infusion in ml/hr? _____

39. A drug is to be administered at 40 mcg in 25 minutes. The patient is receiving 0.12 mg in 1000 ml of D₅W. What is the rate of infusion in ml/hr?   _____

40. A drug is to be administered at 200 ml/hr. The IV set being used is calibrated at 8 drops/ml. What is the drip rate in gtt/min?   _____

41. A physician reduces an IV flow rate to 30 ml/hr. There are 270 ml remaining of the 1000-ml IV bag. The time is 10:30 am. At what time will the infusion be completed?   _____

42. A patient is receiving 1000 ml of NS at 40 ml/ hr. The IV set is calibrated at 60 gtt/ml. What is the flow rate in drops/min?   _____

43. A patient is receiving an IV 1000 cc per 8 hr. When 600 ml have been run in from the 1-L bag, the physician ordered the remainder to be infused over the next 6 hours. The IV set is calibrated at 10 gtt/ml. What is the new flow rate?   _____

44. A patient is to receive 40 mg of medication in 100 ml of D₅W over 60 min. The IV set is calibrated at 15 drops/ml. What is the flow rate in

   a. ml/hr?   _____

   b. gtt/min?   _____

CHAPTER 34

Dilutions

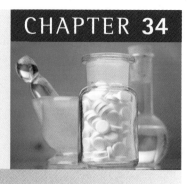

LEARNING OBJECTIVES

After completing this chapter, the student will be able to:

1 Calculate the resulting strength of a solution that has been diluted from a more concentrated strength

2 Calculate the amount of diluent needed to prepare a less concentrated preparation from a more concentrated preparation

KEY TERMS

Dilution: a less concentrated preparation of medication prepared from a more concentrated preparation

Diluent: liquid added to a more concentrated preparation to make a less concentrated preparation

SOMETIMES IT IS NECESSARY to dilute a concentrated solution before dispensing. You may need to calculate the percent concentration of a final volume. You may need to prepare a certain percent dilution and calculate the amount of diluent to add to an available solution.

In the following examples, note the phrases in italics. It is important to distinguish between solutions that are diluted to a certain volume and solutions that have additional solution added to make a final volume.

EXAMPLE

If 500 ml of a 30% solution is *diluted* to 600 ml, what will be the percent strength of the resulting solution?

This problem may be solved in two steps.

1. Calculate how many grams are contained in 500 ml of the 30% solution.

$$\frac{30 \text{ g}}{100 \text{ ml}} = \frac{X}{500 \text{ ml}} \rightarrow X = \frac{30 \text{ g} \times 500 \text{ ml}}{100 \text{ ml}} \rightarrow 150 \text{ g}$$

2. This 150 g is then diluted in 600 ml. To find the percentage strength, calculate how many grams are in 100 ml/ (By definition % is g per 100 ml.)

$$\frac{150 \text{ g}}{600 \text{ ml}} = \frac{X}{100 \text{ ml}} \rightarrow X = \frac{150 \text{ g} \times 100 \text{ ml}}{600 \text{ ml}} \rightarrow 25 \text{ g} \rightarrow 25\% \text{ } answer$$

EXAMPLE

200 ml of a diluent is *added* to 350 ml of a 35% solution. What is the final percent concentration of the diluted solution?

1. Calculate how many grams are contained in 350 ml of 35% solution.

$$\frac{35 \text{ g}}{100 \text{ ml}} = \frac{X}{350 \text{ ml}} \rightarrow X = \frac{35 \text{ g} \times 350 \text{ ml}}{100 \text{ ml}} \rightarrow X = 122.5 \text{ g}$$

Note: The final volume is determined by 200 ml + 350 ml = 550 ml.

2. The 122.5 g is then diluted in 550 ml.

$$\frac{122.5 \text{ g}}{550 \text{ ml}} = \frac{X}{100 \text{ ml}} \rightarrow X = \frac{122.5 \text{ g} \times 100 \text{ ml}}{550 \text{ ml}} \rightarrow 22.27 \text{ g}$$

$\rightarrow$ 22.27% *answer*

EXAMPLE

You *mix together* the following volumes of the same drug: (a) 150 ml of 20% solution; (b) 50 ml of 35% solution, and (c) 20 ml of 50% solution. What is the percent concentration of the final solution after mixing?

1. To solve this problem you need to calculate the total grams from each of the three solutions.

a. $$\frac{20 \text{ g}}{100 \text{ ml}} = \frac{X}{150 \text{ ml}} \rightarrow X = \frac{20 \text{ g} \times 150 \text{ ml}}{100 \text{ ml}} \rightarrow X = 30 \text{ g}$$

b. $$\frac{35 \text{ g}}{100 \text{ ml}} = \frac{X}{50 \text{ ml}} \rightarrow X = \frac{35 \text{ g} \times 50 \text{ ml}}{100 \text{ ml}} \rightarrow X = 17.5 \text{ g}$$

c. $$\frac{50 \text{ g}}{100 \text{ ml}} = \frac{X}{20 \text{ ml}} \rightarrow X = \frac{50 \text{ g} \times 20 \text{ ml}}{100 \text{ ml}} \rightarrow X = 10 \text{ g}$$

Total 57.5 g.

2. The 57.5 g is then diluted in the total volume of the three solutions.

150 ml + 50 ml + 20 ml = 220 ml

$$\frac{57.5 \text{ g}}{220 \text{ m}} = \frac{X}{100 \text{ ml}} \rightarrow X = \frac{35 \text{ g} \times 50 \text{ ml}}{220 \text{ ml}} \rightarrow X = 26.14 \text{ g}$$

$\rightarrow$ 26.14% *answer*

℞ CAPSULE   When calculating a dilution, the amount of drug in a container does not change, but the amount of diluent increases.

EXAMPLE

You are to prepare as much 40% dextrose solution as you can from 200 ml of 70% dextrose solution. How many ml of water do you need to add to the 70% dextrose solution?

1. Calculate how many grams of dextrose is contained in the 200 ml of 70% dextrose solution.

$$\frac{70 \text{ g}}{100 \text{ ml}} = \frac{X}{200 \text{ ml}} \;\rightarrow\; X = \frac{70 \text{ g} \times 200 \text{ ml}}{100 \text{ ml}} \;\rightarrow\; X = 140 \text{ g}$$

2. 140 g is available to prepare 40% dextrose solution. Calculate how many ml will be compounded.

$$\frac{40 \text{ g}}{100 \text{ ml}} = \frac{140 \text{ g}}{X} \;\rightarrow\; X = \frac{140 \text{ g} \times 100 \text{ ml}}{40 \text{ g}}$$

$$\rightarrow X = 350 \text{ ml final solution}$$

3. To find the volume of water required:

Final volume − volume of 70% dextrose solution

350 ml − 200 ml = 150 ml water *answer*

PRACTICE PROBLEMS

STUDENT NAME _____

DATE _____ COURSE NUMBER _____

1. You have 200 ml of a 30% solution. You dilute the solution to 600 ml. What is the percent strength of the final solution? _____

2. What is the percentage strength of a solution that is made by adding 200 ml of purified water to 600 ml of a 25% solution? _____

3. You dilute 50 ml of an 8% solution to 500 ml. What is the percentage strength of the resulting solution? _____

4. A technician has been given 100 ml of a 10% acetic acid solution. The pharmacist asked the technician to dilute the solution to 500 ml with sterile water, and then to label the solution. What % should appear on the label? _____

5. A 20% solution has been diluted to 400 ml and is now a 5% solution. What was the beginning volume of the 20% solution? _____

6. You dilute 75 ml of a 30% solution to 500 ml. What is the percentage
    strength of the final solution prepared?   _____

7. A technician has 50 ml of a 0.5% gentian violet solution on hand. What will be the
    final percentage strength if she dilutes this solution to 125 ml with purified water?   _____

8. If 2 ml of a 1:200 solution are to be mixed with water to make a final concentration
    of 1:1000, how much water is needed?   _____

9. You have on hand 200 g of a 40% ointment. This mixture is to be diluted to 320 g
    with a suitable base. What is the % strength of the resulting ointment?   _____

10. You are preparing a TPN with 500 ml of 7.5% Travasol and 500 ml of 50%
    Dextrose Injection. What is the final percent concentration of the Travasol and
    the dextrose in this TPN?   _____

11. A technician is to compound a TPN with 500 ml of 10% Travasol, 250 ml of
    70% Dextrose Injection and 350 ml of sterile water. What is the final concentration
    of the Travasol and the dextrose in the TPN?   _____

12. You have 4 fluid oz. of a 50% solution and you add 500 ml to this solution. What is the percentage strength of the final solution? _____

13. You have 300 ml of a 20% solution of a drug and 400 ml of 5% solution of the same drug. You mix them together. What is the percentage strength of the final solution? _____

14. If you mix 100 ml of a 1:100 solution with 350 ml of a 1:200 solution, what is the percentage strength of the final solution? What is the ratio strength of the final solution? _____

15. If 14 G of petrolatum are added to 25 G of 0.2% hydrocortisone ointment, what will be the final % concentration of hydrocortisone? _____

16. What is the final percentage strength of a solution when 300 ml of 95%, 1000 ml of 70%, and 200 ml of 50% solutions are mixed together? _____

17. 10 cc of a 50% solution is diluted to 100 cc. What is the % concentration of the diluted solution? _____

18. A technician mixes 80 ml of a 5% solution with 10 ml of water. What is the final percentage strength of the solution prepared? _____

19. A TPN is composed of 300 ml of 7.5% Travasol and 250 ml of 10% dextrose. What is the final percentage strength of the Travasol and the dextrose in the prepared TPN?   _____

20. You have on hand 50 ml of 80% dextrose solution and you need to make as much 35% dextrose solution as possible. How much water will you need to add to the 50 ml of 80% dextrose solution?   _____

21. If 50 ml of a 12% solution is diluted to 120 ml, what is the percentage strength of the new solution?   _____

22. On hand in the pharmacy is 500 ml of a 16% solution. The technician is asked to dilute this stock solution to obtain a 5% solution. How many ml of distilled water will be required?   _____

23. How many ml of an 8% Gentian Violet Solution are required to prepare 120 ml of a 1:400 w/v solution?   _____

24. An order is for 60 G of a 3% ointment. On hand is 100 G of a 10% ointment. The 10% ointment must be diluted with petrolatum. How many grams of each ingredient must be used?   _____

25. In the pharmacy is 500 ml of a 75% stock solution. If the technician adds 300 ml to the stock solution, what percentage strength solution is obtained?   _____

26. In the pharmacy are three different percentage strength stock solutions of the same drug. If these are all mixed together, how many ml and what percentage strength solution will result?

    120 ml of 75%

    54 ml of 10%   _____

    20 ml of 8%

27. A 1:1000 w/v solution is required by a patient. On hand in the pharmacy is 20 ml of a 1:250 w/v solution. How many ml of the 1:1000 w/v solution can be made from the stock solution?   _____

28. You mix 500 ml of 7.5% Travasol and 500 ml of 60% dextrose solution and 300 ml of Sterile Water for Injection. What are the percentage strengths of the Travasol and dextrose in the mixed solution?   _____

29. If 200 ml of Sterile Water for Injection is added to 85 ml of an 80% stock solution, what is the percentage strength of the resulting solution?   _____

30. If 700 ml of Sterile Water for Injection is added to 10 ml of a 10% stock solution, what is the ratio strength of the resulting solution?   _____

31. 20 ml of a 1:1000 w/v stock solution is diluted to 200 ml with Sterile Water for Injection. What is the ratio strength of the diluted solution?   _____

32. An order is received for 90 G of a 0.2% ointment. Available in the pharmacy is a 2.5% ointment that can be diluted with petrolatum. How many grams of the 2.5% ointment and how many grams of the petrolatum will be needed?   _____

33. A physician orders 75 ml of a solution that contains 20 G of the required drug. The stock solution in the pharmacy is a 33% solution. How many ml of the stock solution should be diluted with purified water to obtain the strength of the solution ordered by the physician?   _____

34. A technician is asked to prepare a 42% solution. In stock in the pharmacy is 350 ml of a 55% solution. How many ml can the technician prepare if she uses all the stock solution?   _____

35. The total volume of the additives for a TPN is 125 ml. The TPN also contains 500 ml of 7.5% Travasol with lytes and 500 ml of 45% dextrose solution. What is the final % concentration of the Travasol and dextrose when the TPN is completed?   _____

36. A 1:5000 w/v solution is required to fill an order. On hand in the pharmacy is a 1:200 w/v solution. If the order is for 300 ml, how many ml of the stock solution will be needed?   _____

37. A physician orders a liter of half strength Dakin's Solution. On hand in the pharmacy is full strength Dakin's Solution (0.5% sodium hypochlorite solution). How many ml of the stock solution are needed?   _____

38. Available in the pharmacy is 236 ml of a 10% Povidone-Iodine wash concentrate. The physician orders a diluted wash. If 240 ml of 1% Povidone-Iodine wash is ordered, how many ml of the 10% will be needed?   _____

39. 250 ml of a 26.75% solution must be diluted to an 18% solution before administration. How many ml of water must be added?   _____

40. 400 ml of SWFI is added to 1 liter of normal saline solution. What is the percentage strength of the resulting solution?   _____

41. A technician is asked to make 3 L of a 1:80 solution from a 1:40 stock solution. How many ml of the stock solution are needed?   _____

42. You have on hand a 2% stock solution. How many ml of stock solution are needed to prepare 0.4 L of a 1% solution?   _____

43. If 400 ml of a 20% solution is added to 2.5 L of sterile water, what is the percent strength of the final solution?   _____

44. What is the percent strength of the final solution when the following alcohol strengths are mixed together? 300 ml 95%, 1000 ml 70%, and 200 ml 50 %
    Hint: Round your number.   _____

CHAPTER 35

Alligations

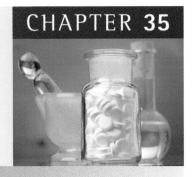

LEARNING OBJECTIVES

After completing this chapter, the student will be able to:

1 Describe how to set up an alligation

2 Use alligation to determine how to prepare a concentration of an ingredient from two concentrations of the same ingredient when the desired concentration is in between the concentrations of the two available concentrations

KEY TERMS

Alligation: type of calculation to determine how much of two concentrations of the same ingredient are needed to prepare a concentration that is in between

Part: relative amount of an ingredient

IF A CERTAIN PERCENTAGE STRENGTH SOLUTION is needed but not available, a technician can prepare it by mixing together a stronger percentage strength solution and a weaker percentage strength solution in appropriate proportions to achieve the desired strength.

All concentrations must be in a percentage form and the strength of the desired solution must lie between the stronger and weaker solutions available. If the concentration is not expressed in the percentage form, it must be converted to the percentage form. For example, a solution strength expressed as 1:200 must be converted to a percentage.

$$\rightarrow \frac{1}{200} \times 100 = 0.5\%$$

These types of calculations are known as alligations, and they are set up using a layout similar to a tic-tac-toe board.

Higher % Strength Solution ↘		Number of Parts of Higher % Solution
minus	Required % Strength Solution ↗ ↘	
Lower % Strength Solution	minus	Number of Parts of Lower % Solution

- The higher % strength is always placed in the upper left box.

- The lower % strength is always placed in the lower left box.

- The required % strength is always placed in the center box.

- The higher % strength minus the required % strength equals the number of parts of lower % strength solution needed.

- The required % strength minus the lower % strength equals the number of parts of higher % strength solution needed.

- The *total parts* are equal to the sum of the higher % and lower % parts.

- The volume of higher % strength solution needed is determined by dividing the number of parts of higher % strength solution by the total parts and then multiplying by the final volume required.

- Similarily, the volume of lower % strength solution needed is determined by dividing the number of parts of lower % strength solution by the total parts and then multiplying by the final volume required.

EXAMPLE

You receive an order for 500 ml of 40% dextrose solution. On hand are stock solutions of 60% dextrose and 25% dextrose. How many ml of each of the stock solutions will you need to prepare this order?

Set up a tic-tac-toe layout.

60%		15 parts
minus ↘	40% ↗ ↘	
minus		
25%		20 parts

Total parts = 35

$\dfrac{15}{35} \times 500 \text{ ml} = 214.3 \text{ ml}$
(round to 214 ml)
of 60% dextrose
solution

$\dfrac{20}{35} \times 500 \text{ ml} = 285.7 \text{ ml}$
(round to 286 ml)
of 25% dextrose
solution

The sum of the volumes for the higher and lower % strengths must equal the final volume.

This method of calculation can also be used when diluting a solution with water. Water is given the value of 0% and is always placed in the lower left box of the tic-tac-toe layout.

> ℞ CAPSULE   When setting up an alligation, remember to place the higher strength in the upper left box and the lower strength in the lower left box.

EXAMPLE

A technician is asked to prepare 350 ml of a 22% boric acid solution from a 50% boric acid solution and purified water. How many ml of 50% solution and water will be needed?

Set up a tic-tac-toe layout.

50%		22 parts
minus	22%	
minus		
0%		28 parts

Total parts = 50

$$\frac{22}{50} \times 350 \text{ ml} = 154 \text{ ml of } 50\% \text{ boric acid solution}$$

$$\frac{28}{50} \times 350 \text{ ml} = 196 \text{ ml of water}$$

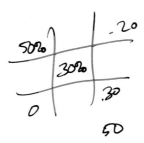

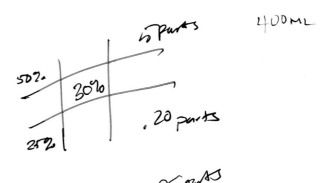

PRACTICE PROBLEMS

STUDENT NAME_____

DATE _____   COURSE NUMBER _____

Round all answers to the nearest whole number unless otherwise directed.

1. Calculate how many ml of 50% dextrose solution and how many ml of water are needed to prepare 4.5 L of a 1% solution.   _____

2. How many ml of a 50% solution and how many ml of a 5% solution are needed to prepare 4 liters of a 10% solution?   _____

3. How many ml of a 15% solution of sodium chloride and ml of water should be used to prepare 1 liter of a 0.9% solution of sodium chloride?   _____

4. How many ml of each of a 20% stock solution and a 30% stock solution will a technician need to make 500 ml of a 28% solution?   _____

5. How many grams of 10% boric acid ointment should be mixed with petrolatum (0%) to prepare 700 G of a 5% boric acid ointment?   _____

6. You have on hand 10% and 3% ammoniated mercury ointment. You need to prepare 450 g of a 5% ointment. How many grams of each of the 10% and the 3% ointment will you need?   _____

7. A technician is to prepare 2.5 liters of a 1:20 solution from a 30% solution and water. How many ml of the 30% solution and water are needed?   _____

8. A TPN order requires 500 ml of $D_{30}W$. You find that you do not have any $D_{30}W$ in stock, you only have $D_{40}W$ and sterile water. How many ml of $D_{40}W$ and sterile water will you need to complete this order?   _____

9. A hospital clinic requests 2 pounds of 2% hydrocortisone ointment. How many grams of 5% hydrocortisone ointment would be diluted with white petrolatum (0%) to prepare this order?   _____

10. How many ml of a 1:400 stock solution and purified water should be used to prepare 4 liters of a 1:2000 solution?

    _____

11. You receive an order for 200 ml of potassium permanganate 1:5000 solution. You have in the pharmacy a 2% potassium permanganate stock solution. How many ml of the stock solution and purified water will you need to compound this prescription?

    _____

12. How many ml of a 16% stock solution are needed to compound 400 ml of a 1:2500 solution?

    _____

13. Calculate how many ml of a 1:2 solution and ml of water are needed to prepare 50 ml of a 15% solution.

    _____

14. A technician has on hand 70% dextrose stock solution and 40% dextrose stock solution. She is to prepare 1000 ml of 45% dextrose solution. How many ml of each of the stock solutions will she need?

    _____

15. You are to prepare 350 ml of a 1:50 solution from 1:10 and 1:1000 stock solutions. How many ml of each of the stock solutions do you need?   _____

16. Calculate how many ml of a 30% stock solution and ml of a 85% stock solution are needed to prepare 3 liters of 60% solution.   _____

17. A physician orders 250 g of a 5% ointment. On hand in the pharmacy are 2% and 10% stock ointments. How many grams of each of the stock ointments are needed to prepare the order?   _____

18. An order calls for 16 fl. oz. of a 20% solution. On hand are stock solutions of 80% and 8%. How many ml of each of the stock solutions are needed to fill the order?   _____

19. A technician is asked to prepare a prescription for 10 fl. oz. of a 35% solution. In stock is a 50% solution. How many ml of the 50% stock solution and how many ml of purified water are needed to prepare the prescription?   _____

20. A prescription is written for 4 fl. oz. of a 7.5% solution. How many fl. oz. each of a 10% stock solution and purified water will be needed to compound this prescription? _____

21. In the pharmacy are two stock solutions 50% and 20%. How many ml of each solution will be needed to prepare 800 ml of a 33% solution? _____

22. Stock solutions of 27% and 31% are available in the pharmacy. How many ml of each stock solution are needed to prepare 2 liters of a 29% solution? _____

23. Two very dilute stock solutions are available to prepare 60 ml of a 1:1000 w/v solution. The two stock solutions are 1:200 w/v and 1:2000 w/v. How many ml of each will be required? _____

24. Hydrogen peroxide stock solution is available in a 3.5% strength. How many ml of stock solution and water will be needed to prepare 120 ml of a 2.5% solution? _____

25. The technician is asked to prepare 2.5 L of D₅W from a 45% dextrose solution and SWFI. How many ml of each will be needed?   _____

26. An order is received for 60 G of a 1% ointment. Available in the pharmacy is 100 G of 2.5% ointment. How many grams of the 2.5% ointment and petrolatum (used for dilution of the ointment) will be required?   _____

27. A pint of 4% solution is ordered. On hand are 1% and 6% stock solutions. How many fluid ounces of each will be needed to fill the prescription?   _____

28. An order is received for 2 quarts of a 14% solution. Purified water and a 20% solution are to be used for the preparation. How many fluid ounces of each are needed?   _____

29. A technician is to prepare 500 ml of a 1:400 w/v solution from a 1% solution and purified water. How many ml of each will be needed?   _____

30. From two stock solutions, 18% and 42%, you are to prepare 1.5 L of a 34% solution. How many ml of each of the stock solutions do you need?   _____

31. An order for 60 ml of a 1% topical liquid is to be prepared from a 5% solution and purified water. How many ml of each are needed?   _____

32. An order for 6 liters of 0.9% sodium chloride solution is to be prepared from 23.4% concentrated NaCl solution and Sterile Water for Injection. How many ml of each will be used?   _____

33. Silver Nitrate Topical Solution is available in 25% and 50% stock solutions. An order is received for 30 ml of 30% solution. How many ml of each of the stock solutions will be needed?   _____

34. An order is received for 50 ml of 7.2% solution to be prepared from 4.2% and 8.4% stock solutions. How many ml of each of the stock solutions will be needed?   _____

35. On hand in the pharmacy are two stock solutions, 0.75% and 3%. A prescription is for 15 ml of a 1.5% solution. How many ml of the two stock solutions are required?   _____

36. A technician is to prepare 250 ml of a 40% solution from a 60% stock solution and purified water. How many ml of each are needed?   _____

37. An order reads 30 ml of 0.6% solution. Available in the pharmacy are two stock solutions, 0.4% and 5%. How many ml of each stock solution will be used to fill the order?   _____

38. The pharmacy has run out of 500 ml bags of 1/2 NS. The technician is to use 0.9% sodium chloride solution and Sterile Water for Injection to make a 500 ml bag of 1/2 NS. How many ml of NS and SWFI will she need?   _____

39. The technician is to prepare 800 G of a 3% ointment. In the pharmacy is a
     10% ointment and petrolatum. How many grams of the stock ointment and
     petrolatum will he or she weigh out?   _____

40. A liter of 1/3 NS is to be prepared from 23.4% concentrated sodium chloride
     solution and Sterile Water for Injection. How many ml of each are to be used?   _____

41. On hand in the pharmacy is concentrated NaCl 23.4%. The technician is required to
     prepare 50 ml of 14.6% NaCl solution. How many ml of 23.4% and water are needed?   _____

42. An order calls for 200 ml of Dakins Solution (0.125% sodium hypochlorite).
     A 0.5% stock solution is available. How many ml of the stock solution and
     water will be needed to fill the order?   _____

43. Three hundred milliliters (300 ml) of a 3% irrigation solution is ordered. The stock solution in the pharmacy is a 3.3% solution. How many ml of stock solution and water will be needed?   _____

44. On hand are two stock solutions, 10% and 5%. The technician is to prepare 60 ml of 7.5% solution using both stock solutions. How many ml of each will be required?   _____

45. A physician orders 2 ml of a 0.12% solution. In the pharmacy is a 1% solution. How many ml of the stock solution and water are needed to prepare the order? Do not round this answer.   _____

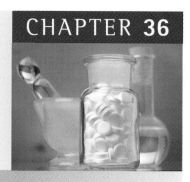

Parenteral Nutrition Calculations

LEARNING OBJECTIVES

After completing this chapter, the student will be able to:

1 Define the terms *parenteral nutrition solution* and *hyperalimentation solution*

2 Explain the difference between a TPN and a PPN

3 Identify possible base solutions used in TPNs and PPNs

4 Identify possible additives used in TPNs and PPNs

5 Perform calculations to determine the amounts of ingredients needed to prepare TPNs and PPNs

KEY TERMS

Parenteral nutrition solution: solution to provide nutrition to patients via IV (also known as hyperalimentation solution)

Hyperalimentation solution: solution to provide nutrition to patients via IV (also known as parenteral nutrition solution)

TPN: total parenteral nutrition solution that provides all necessary nutrients for a patient

PPN: partial parenteral nutrition solution that provides some nutrients for a patient who is also receiving nutrition by another type of feeding

Base solution: for a TPN or PPN, can consist of carbohydrates, proteins, or essential fatty acid emulsions

Additives: for a TPN or PPN, can consist of electrolytes, vitamins, trace elements, insulin, and/or other additives as prescribed to be include in the TPN or PPN

PARENTERAL NUTRITION SOLUTIONS (also known as hyperalimentation solutions) are a means of providing nutrition to patients via IV, either to replace or maintain essential nutrients.

There are two main types of parenteral nutrition solutions:

- Total Parenteral Nutrition (TPN): These solutions provide all nutrients for a patient.

- Partial Parenteral Nutrition (PPN): These solutions provide some nutrients parenterally combined with other types of feeding such as enteral and/or oral feeding.

Some indications for parenteral nutrition include: gastrointestinal disease, malnutrition, major organ failure, major surgery, and cancer.

A TPN consists of a base solution and additives.

Base Solution

1. Carbohydrates obtained from high concentration dextrose solutions 10% to 70%.

2. Proteins obtained from amino acids solutions 3.5% to 15% (brand names such as Travasol and Aminosyn).

3. Essential fatty acids from fat emulsions 10% and 20%.

> **R̥ CAPSULE**   The fat emulsion is not always admixed into the TPN. If it is included, the TPN is known as a 3-in-1 TPN. Fat emulsions may be administered to the patient as a separate infusion.

Additives

1. Electrolytes such as sodium chloride, potassium chloride, calcium gluconate, magnesium sulfate, sodium acetate, and potassium phosphates. Electrolytes are prescribed according to patient needs as determined from blood levels.

> **R̥ CAPSULE**   Care must be taken when adding a calcium and a phosphate to a TPN. In certain concentrations, these electrolytes are incompatible and a precipitate will form. To minimize this problem, the phosphate is added first to the TPN to allow for dilution of the phosphate and the calcium is added last after all other additives.

2. Vitamins

3. Trace elements

4. Insulin

5. Other additives as prescribed

Typically a TPN will have 6 to 10 additives mixed with the base solution. There is, therefore, a large number of calculations to be performed so great care must be taken and a check by a second person is desirable.

Physicians may prescribe TPNs in a variety of ways:

■ Standard formulation: This is a TPN formula developed by the institution, and physicians use this if appropriate for their patient's needs.

■ Patient specific: Amino acids, dextrose, and lipids are ordered as grams, and/or grams per kilogram of body weight; electrolytes are ordered as milliequivalents (mEq) or millimoles (mM), and/or mEq or mM per kilogram of body weight.

Calculations for TPN additives may be performed using the ratio and proportion method described earlier in this text.

EXAMPLE

Dose required is KCl 30 mEq. The concentration available is 2 mEq/ml.

Set up a ratio and proportion:

$$\frac{2 \text{ mEq}}{1 \text{ ml}} = \frac{30 \text{ mEq}}{X} \quad \rightarrow \quad \frac{X \times \cancel{2 \text{ mEq}}}{\cancel{2 \text{ mEq}}} = \frac{1 \text{ ml} \times 30 \cancel{\text{ mEq}}}{2 \cancel{\text{ mEq}}}$$

$\rightarrow$ X = 15 ml *answer*

EXAMPLE

The following TPN is ordered. Calculate the final % concentrations of Travasol and dextrose in the completed TPN.

Base Solutions

Travasol	500 ml of 5%
Dextrose	900 ml of 45%

Additives

Potassium chloride	46 ml
Magnesium sulfate	6 ml
MVI	10 ml
Calcium gluconate	20 ml

Step 1: Calculate the grams of Travasol and dextrose in the base solutions.

Set up ratio and proportion problems.

Travasol

$$5\% = 5 \text{ g in } 100 \text{ ml}$$

$$\frac{5 \text{ g}}{100 \text{ ml}} = \frac{X}{500 \text{ ml}} \quad \rightarrow \quad X = \frac{5 \text{ g} \times 500 \cancel{\text{ ml}}}{100 \cancel{\text{ ml}}}$$

$$\rightarrow \quad = 25 \text{ g Travasol}$$

Dextrose

$$45\% = 45 \text{ g in } 100 \text{ ml}$$

$$\frac{45 \text{ g}}{100 \text{ ml}} = \frac{X}{900 \text{ ml}} \quad \rightarrow \quad X = \frac{45 \text{ g} \times 900 \cancel{\text{ ml}}}{100 \cancel{\text{ ml}}}$$

$$\rightarrow \quad = 405 \text{ g Dextrose}$$

Step 2: Add together the ml of Travasol and dextrose and the additives in the TPN.

Total $\rightarrow$ 1482 ml

Step 3:   Calculate the % concentrations of Travasol and dextrose in the total ml.

Remember % is grams per 100 ml.s

Set up ratio and proportion problems to calculate number of grams in 100 ml.

Travasol

$$\frac{25 \text{ g}}{1482 \text{ ml}} = \frac{X}{100 \text{ ml}} \;\rightarrow\; X = \frac{25 \text{ g} \times 100 \text{ ml}}{1482 \text{ ml}}$$

$$\rightarrow\quad = 1.69 \text{ g}$$

$$\rightarrow\quad = 1.69\% \text{ Travasol} \quad answer$$

Dextrose

$$\frac{405 \text{ g}}{1482 \text{ ml}} = \frac{X}{100 \text{ ml}} \;\rightarrow\; X = \frac{405 \text{ g} \times 100 \text{ ml}}{1482 \text{ ml}}$$

$$\rightarrow\quad = 27.33 \text{ g}$$

$$\rightarrow\quad = 27.33\% \text{ dextrose} \quad answer$$

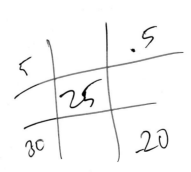

PRACTICE PROBLEMS

STUDENT NAME_____

DATE _____ COURSE NUMBER _____

For all the TPN calculations in this section, use the following concentrations:

Potassium chloride	2 mEq/ml	
Sodium chloride	14.6%	2.5 mEq/ml
Calcium gluconate	10%	4.65 mEq/10 ml
Magnesium sulfate	50%	40.6 mEq/10 ml
Sodium acetate	2 mEq/ml	
Sodium phosphate	45 mM/15 ml	60 mEq/15 ml
Potassium acetate	19.6%	2 mEq/ml
Potassium phosphate	15 mM/5 ml	4.4 mEq/ml
Humulin R insulin	100 units/ml	
Vitamin C	250 mg/2 ml	

For the following TPN formulas, No. 1 through No. 8, calculate the ml required for each additive.

EXAMPLE

TPN No. 1: sodium chloride ordered is 25 mEq.

Concentration of sodium chloride available = 2.5 mEq/ml. (Remember, you must use the same units.)

Set up a ratio and proportion:

$$\frac{2.5 \text{ mEq}}{1 \text{ ml}} = \frac{25 \text{ mEq}}{X} \rightarrow \frac{X \times \cancel{2.5 \text{ mEq}}}{\cancel{2.5 \text{ mEq}}} = \frac{1 \text{ ml} \times 25 \cancel{\text{ mEq}}}{2.5 \cancel{\text{ mEq}}}$$

$\rightarrow X = 10 \text{ ml}$ *answer*

Base Solutions	No. 1	No. 2	No. 3	No. 4
Travasol 7.5 % with lytes	500 ml		500 ml	500 ml
Travasol 10 % without lytes		500 ml		
Dextrose 70 %	500 ml	350 ml	300 ml	500 ml
Sterile Water for Injection		250 ml	200 ml	
Rate ml/hr	60 ml/hr	60 ml/hr	60 ml/hr	60 ml/hr

Additives	No. 1	No. 2	No. 3	No. 4
Sodium chloride	25 mEq	12 mEq	15 mEq	20 mEq
Potassium chloride	30 mEq	20 mEq	10 mEq	14 mEq
Magnesium sulfate	12 mEq	20 mEq	500 mg	2 G
Potassium phosphates	22 mEq	9 mM	12 mM	17.6 mEq
Calcium gluconate	56 mEq	1 G	1.5 G	24 mEq
MVI-12 10 ml/vial	10 ml	10 ml	10 ml	10 ml
Trace elements	5 ml	5 ml	5 ml	5 ml
Vitamin C	125 mg	500 mg	625 mg	750 mg
Humulin R insulin	55 units	60 units	80 units	95 units
Folic acid (5 mg/ml)	2.5 mg	5 mg	6.25 mg	3.75 mg
Sodium acetate	40 mEq	35 mEq	10 mEq	14 mEq
Potassium acetate	14 mEq	20 mEq	25 mEq	8 mEq
Sodium phosphates	4 mEq	20 mEq	8 mEq	12 mM

Show your work here.

Show your work here.

5. *A patient is ordered the following TPN. Calculate the milliliters needed for each additive. (Use the concentrations provided previously.)*

Base Solutions: 7.5% Travasol   500 ml

                   60% Dextrose solution   500 ml

Additives: Potassium chloride   84 mEq

                   Sodium chloride   60 mEq

                   Magnesium sulfate   8 mEq

                   Trace elements   5 ml

                   Sodium acetate   20 mEq

                   Humulin R insulin   54 units

                   Calcium gluconate   2.5 G

What are the final % concentrations of Travasol and dextrose in the TPN?

6. *The following TPN is ordered for a patient whose weight is 20 kg. Calculate the milliliters needed for each additive.*

| Base Solutions: | 5% Travasol | 250 ml |
| | 20% Dextrose solution | 150 ml |

Additives:	Sodium chloride	3 mEq/kg
	Potassium chloride	2.5 mEq/kg
	Calcium gluconate	1.5 mEq/kg
	Magnesium sulfate	0.5 mEq/kg
	Potassium phosphate	1 mMol/kg

What are the % concentrations of the Travasol and the dextrose in the completed TPN?

7. *Calculate the milliliters needed for each additive in the following TPN.*

Base Solutions:	10% Travasol	1000 ml
	50% Dextrose solution	1000 ml
	Sterile Water for Injection	500 ml

Additives:	Potassium chloride	120 mEq
	Sodium chloride	86 mEq
	Magnesium sulfate	24 mEq
	Calcium gluconate	9 mEq
	Trace elements	5 ml
	MVI	10 ml
	Potassium phosphate	40 mMol
	Humulin R insulin	68 units

Calculate the final % strengths of the base solutions in the compounded TPN.

8. *A TPN is to be compounded with the following medications. Calculate the milliliters required for each additive.*

| Base Solutions: | 8.5% Aminosyn | 550 ml |
| | 60% Dextrose solution | 500 ml |

Additives:	Potassium chloride	140 mEq
	Sodium chloride	105 mEq
	Magnesium sulfate	1 G
	Calcium gluconate	2 G
	Potassium phosphate	13.2 mEq
	Vitamin C	750 mg

What are the final % concentrations of the Aminosyn and the dextrose in the TPN?

Dosage Calculations from Medication Labels

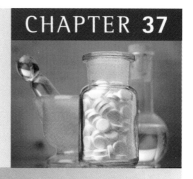

LEARNING OBJECTIVES

After completing this chapter, the student will be able to:

1 Calculate the volume of a drug that is needed to deliver a specific dose of a medication using information provided on the manufacturer's label

2 Describe how powdered medications that require reconstitution are prepared to deliver the prescribed dose of a medication

KEY TERM

Reconstitution: adding a specified amount of diluent to a powdered drug preparation before administration

IN THE PRACTICE OF PHARMACY, quantities needed are calculated from labeled vials of medication.

Using the labels provided, calculate the milliliters needed for the following dosages.

You may set up ratio and proportion equations, but the aim of this chapter is for you to do the calculations with confidence in your head or with the aid of a calculator.

Note: Pfizerpen inj, Cytarabine inj, and Zithromax inj are powdered medications that require reconstitution. Use the concentrations obtained after reconstitution as indicated on the labels. (Add 5 ml SWI to 100 mg Cytarabine inj.) Where more than one concentration can be obtained, give answers for all concentrations, indicating which concentration was used for your answers.

EXAMPLE

Calculate from the label provided the number of ml needed for the prescribed dose.

1. 500 mg calcium gluconate

   Remember: the units must match.

   From the label, the concentration to use is 10%.

   10% = 10 g in 100 ml

   Reduce to g/ml   →   1 g/10 ml   →   0.1 g/ml

   Convert 0.1 g to mg   →   100 mg/ml

   Can set up a ratio and proportion equation, if necessary:

   $$\frac{100 \text{ mg}}{1 \text{ ml}} = \frac{500 \text{ mg}}{X} \qquad X = \frac{500 \text{ mg}}{100 \text{ mg}}$$

   $$= 5 \text{ ml} \quad \textit{answer}$$

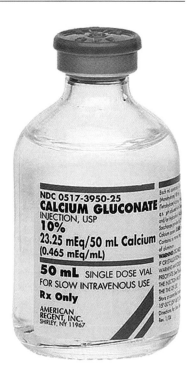

2. 9.3 mEq calcium gluconate

   Remember: the units must match.

   From the label, the concentration to use is 0.465 mEq/ml.

   Set up ratio and proportion, if necessary.

   $$\frac{0.465 \text{ mEq}}{1 \text{ ml}} = \frac{9.3 \text{ mEq}}{X} \qquad X = \frac{9.3 \text{ mEq}}{0.465 \text{ mEq}}$$

   $$= 20 \text{ ml} \quad \textit{answer}$$

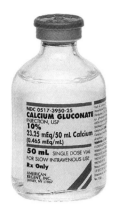
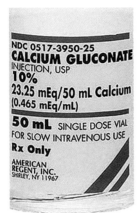

1. CALCIUM GLUCONATE INJ   210 mg

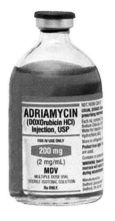
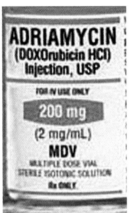

2. ADRIAMYCIN INJ   33 mg

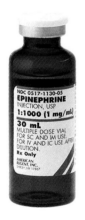
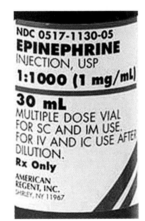

3. EPINEPHRINE INJ   0.5 mg

4. GENTAMICIN INJ   175 mg

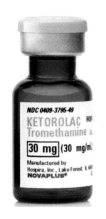

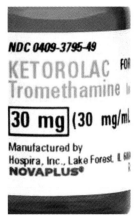

5. KETOROLAC INJ   15 mg

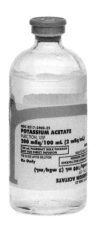

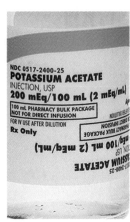

6. POTASSIUM ACETATE INJ   10 mEq

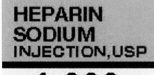

7. HEPARIN INJ   17,500 units

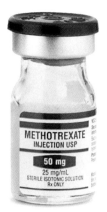

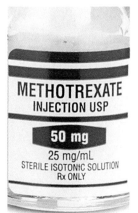

8. METHOTREXATE INJ   720 mg

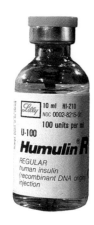 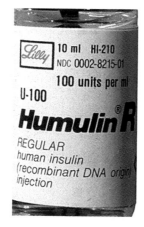

9. HUMULIN R INJ 32 units

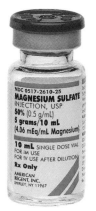 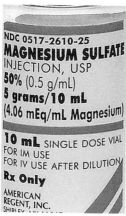

10. MAGNESIUM SULFATE INJ 6 G

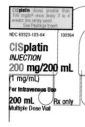

11. CISPLATIN INJ 67.5 mg

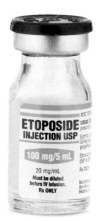 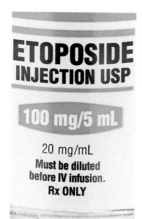

12. ETOPOSIDE INJ 75 mg

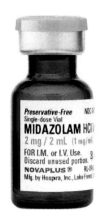
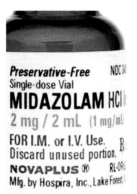

13. MIDAZOLAM INJ   2 mg

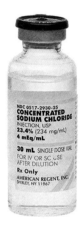
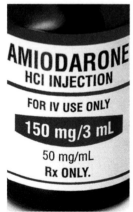

14. SODIUM CHLORIDE INJ   2.3 G

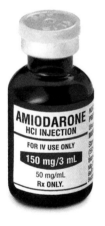

15. AMIODARONE INJ   1000 mg

16. GENTAMICIN PED INJ   30 mg

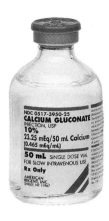

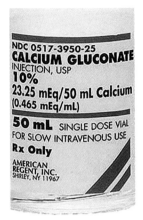

17. CALCIUM GLUCONATE INJ   1.3 G

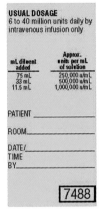

18. PFIZERPEN INJ   3.5 mu

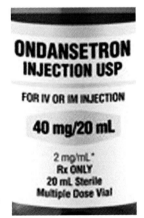

19. ONDANSETRON INJ   13.5 mg

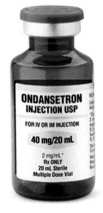

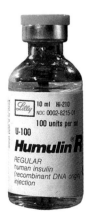

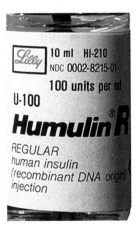

20. HUMULIN R INJ   54 units

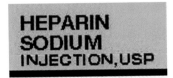

21.   HEPARIN INJ   450 units

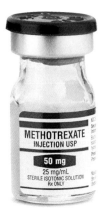
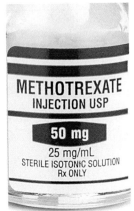

22.   METHOTREXATE INJ   69 mg

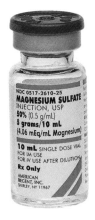
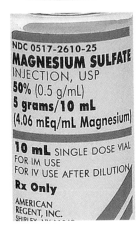

23.   MAGNESIUM SULFATE INJ   40 mEq

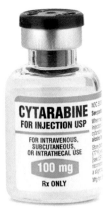
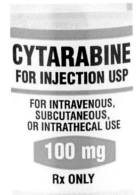

24.   CYTARABINE INJ   98 mg

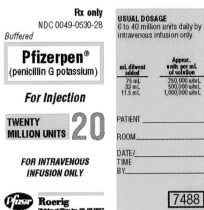
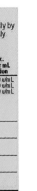

25. PFIZERPEN INJ   6,000,000 units

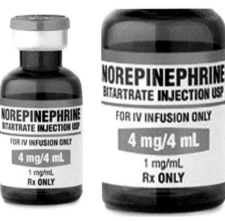

26. NOREPINEPHRINE INJ   32 mg

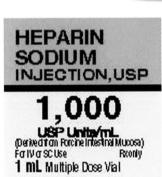

27. HEPARIN INJ   5000 units

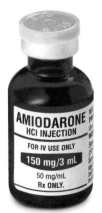
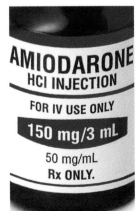

28. AMIODARONE INJ   125 mg

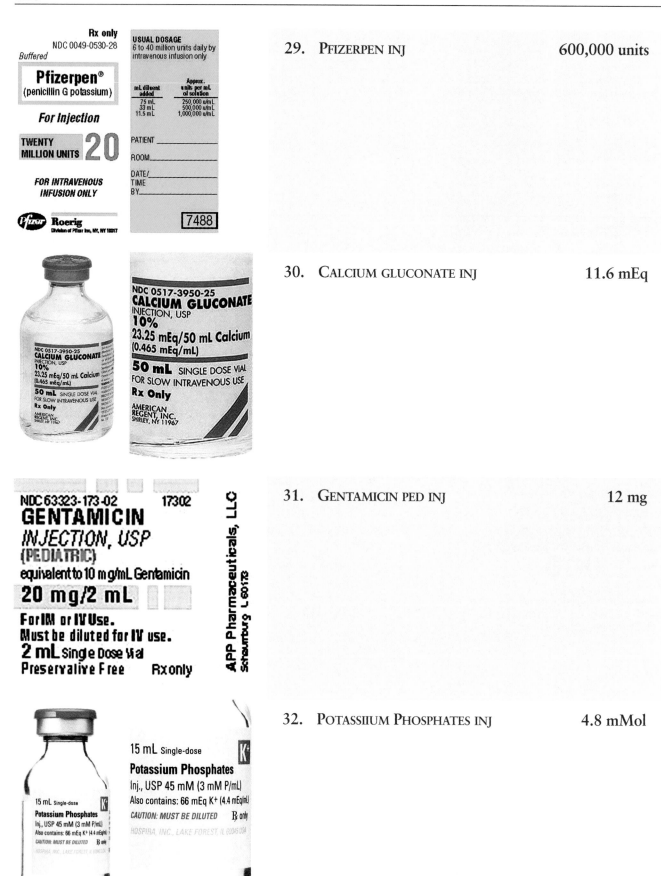

29. PFIZERPEN INJ   600,000 units

30. CALCIUM GLUCONATE INJ   11.6 mEq

31. GENTAMICIN PED INJ   12 mg

32. POTASSIIUM PHOSPHATES INJ   4.8 mMol

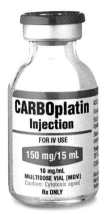
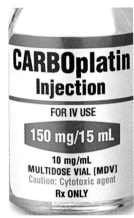

33. CARBOPLATIN INJ   910 mg

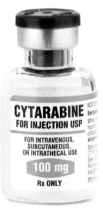
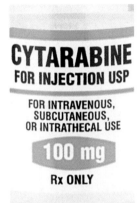

34. CYTARABINE INJ   25 mg

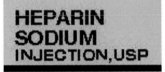

35. HEPARIN INJ   1080 units

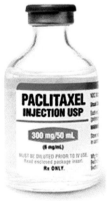
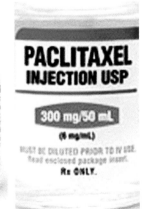

36. PACLITAXEL INJ   500 mg

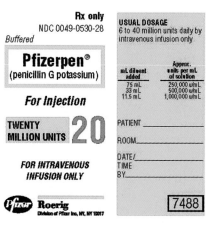

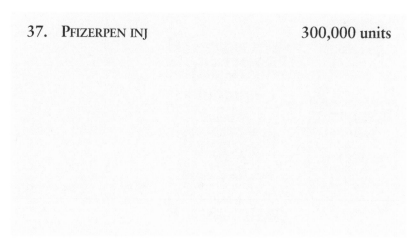

37. PFIZERPEN INJ   300,000 units

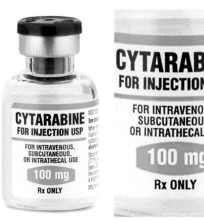

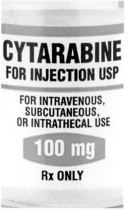

38. CYTARABINE INJ   1500 mg

39. EPINEPHRINE INJ   0.15 mg

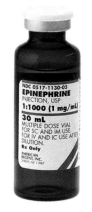

40. GENTAMICIN INJ   240 mg

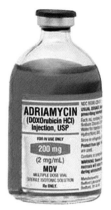
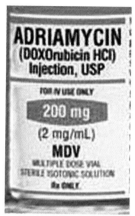

41.   ADRIAMYCIN INJ   85 mg

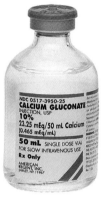
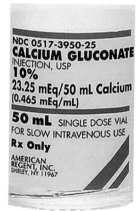

42.   CALCIUM GLUCONATE INJ   270 mg

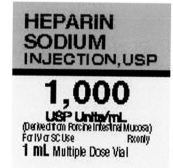

43.   HEPARIN INJ   900 units

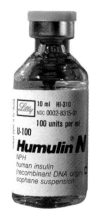
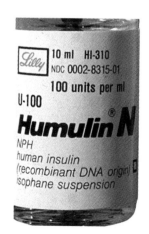

44.   HUMULIN N INJ   78 units

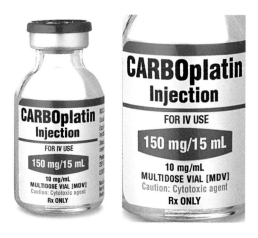

45.   CARBOPLATIN INJ   420 mg

46.   ZITHROMAX INJ   275 mg

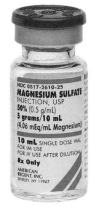
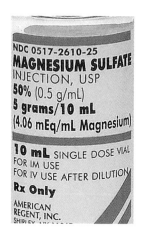

47.   MAGNESIUM SULFATE INJ   3 mEq

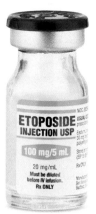
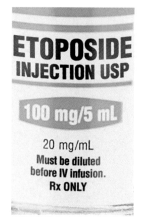

48.   ETOPOSIDE INJ   300 mg

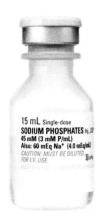

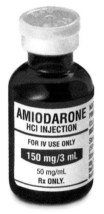

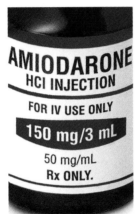

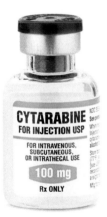

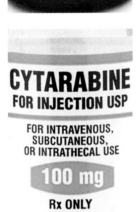

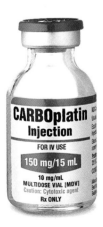

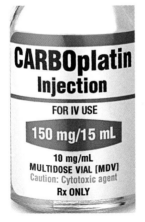

49. SODIUM PHOSPHATES INJ   6 mMol

50. AMIODARONE INJ   360 mg

51. CYTARABINE INJ   500 mg

52. CARBOPLATIN INJ   120 mg

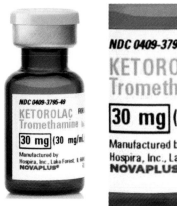
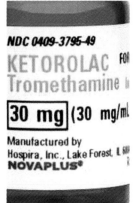

53.   KETOROLAC INJ   30 mg

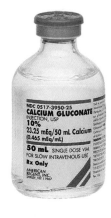
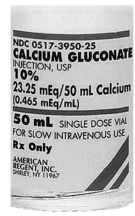

54.   CALCIUM GLUCONATE INJ   1300 mg

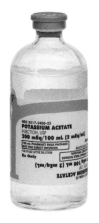
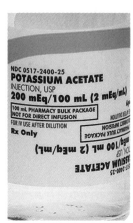

55.   POTASSIUM ACETATE INJ   30 mEq

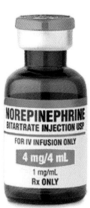
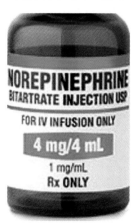

56.   NOREPINEPHRINE INJ   4 mg

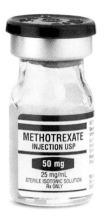
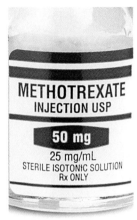

57. METHOTREXATE INJ   85 mg

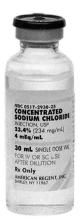
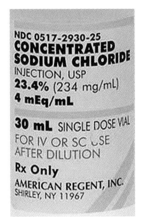

58. PFIZERPEN INJ   560,000 units

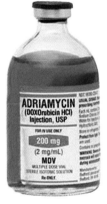
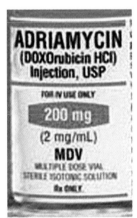

59. ADRIAMYCIN INJ   19 mg

60. SODIUM CHLORIDE INJ   4 mEq

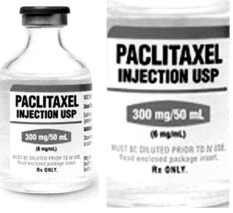

61. HEPARIN INJ   1500 units

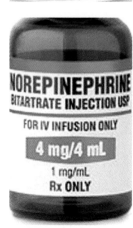
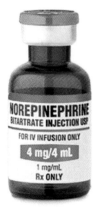

62. PACLITAXEL INJ   227 mg

63. NOREPINEPHRINE INJ   12 mg

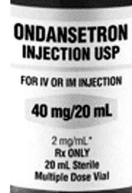
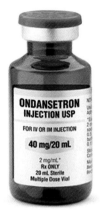

64. ONDANSETRON INJ   4 mg

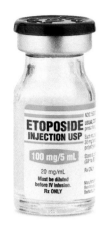
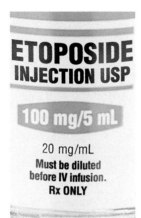

65. ETOPOSIDE INJ   120 mg

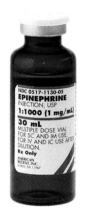
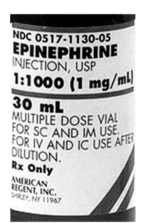

66. EPINEPHRINE INJ   100 mcg

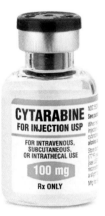
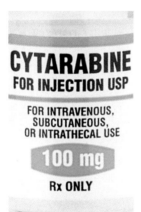

67. CYTARABINE INJ   325 mg

68. ZITHROMAX INJ   250 mg

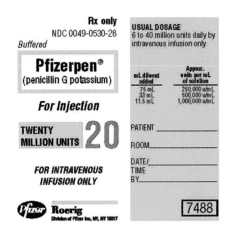

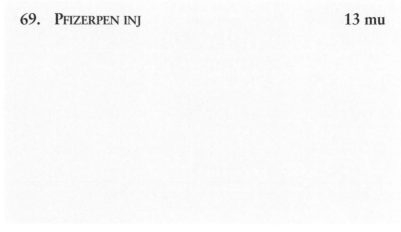

69. PFIZERPEN INJ   13 mu

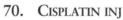

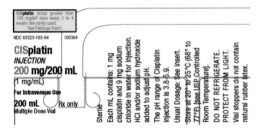

70. CISPLATIN INJ   36 mg

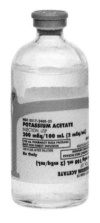

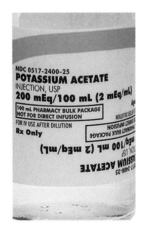

71. POTASSIUM ACETATE INJ   85 mEq

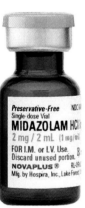

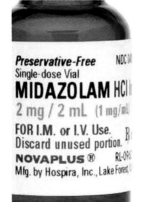

72. MIDAZOLAM INJ   3.5 mg

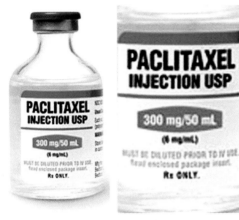

73. PACLITAXEL INJ   210 mg

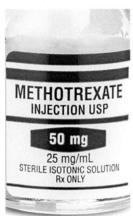

74. METHOTREXATE INJ   145 mg

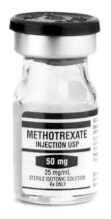
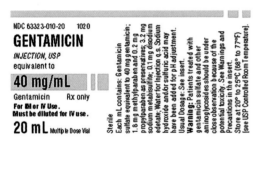

75. GENTAMICIN INJ   102 mg

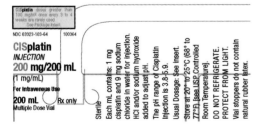

76. CISPLATIN INJ   98 mg

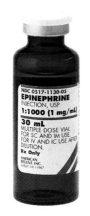
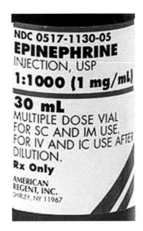

77. EPINEPHRINE INJ   2.5 mg

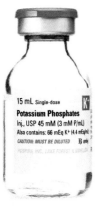
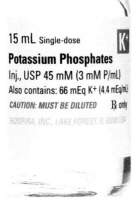

78. POTASSIUM PHOSPHATES   9.6 mMol

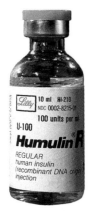
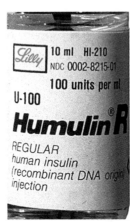

79. HUMULIN R INJ   97 units

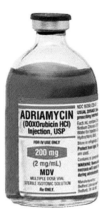
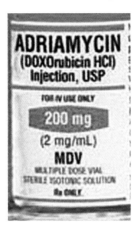

80. ADRIAMYCIN INJ   120 mg

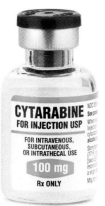

HEPARIN SODIUM INJECTION, USP

1,000
USP Units/mL
(Derived from Porcine Intestinal Mucosa)
For IV or SC Use   Rx only
1 mL Multiple Dose Vial

81. HEPARIN INJ   7400 units

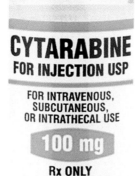

CYTARABINE FOR INJECTION USP

FOR INTRAVENOUS, SUBCUTANEOUS, OR INTRATHECAL USE

100 mg

Rx ONLY

82. CYTARABINE INJ   105 mg

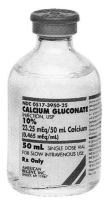

NDC 0517-3950-25
CALCIUM GLUCONATE
INJECTION, USP
10%
23.25 mEq/50 mL Calcium
(0.465 mEq/mL)
50 mL SINGLE DOSE VIAL
FOR SLOW INTRAVENOUS USE
Rx Only
AMERICAN REGENT, INC.
SHIRLEY, NY 11967

83. CALCIUM GLUCONATE INJ   800 mg

Store at or below 86°F (30°C)

DOSAGE AND USE
See accompanying prescribing information.

Constitute to 100 mg/mL* with
4.8 mL of Sterile Water For Injection.

Must be further diluted before use.
For appropriate diluents and storage
recommendations, refer to prescribing information.

*Each mL contains azithromycin dihydrate
equivalent to 100 mg of azithromycin,
76.9 mg of citric acid, and sodium hydroxide
for pH adjustment.

Rx only

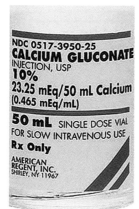

NDC 0069-3150-83
Zithromax®
(azithromycin for injection)

For I.V. infusion only
STERILE
equivalent to
500 mg
of azithromycin
Distributed by
Pfizer Labs
Division of Pfizer Inc, NY, NY 10017

84. ZITHROMAX INJ   500 mg

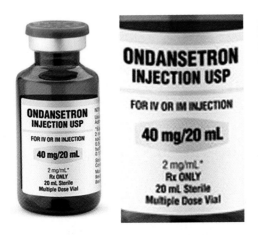

85.   ONDANSETRON INJ   24 mg

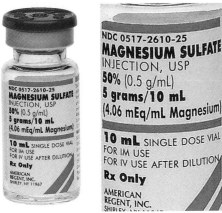

86.   MAGNESIUM SULFATE INJ   2 G

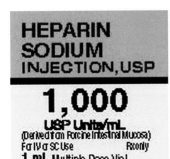

87.   HEPARIN INJ   4500 units

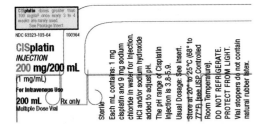

88.   CISPLATIN INJ   16 mg

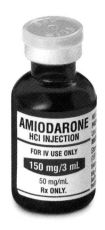
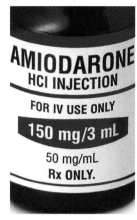

89. AMIODARONE INJ   1300 mg

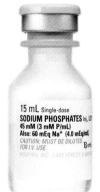

90. PFIZERPEN INJ   1.5 mu

91. SODIUM PHOSPHATES INJ   12 mMol

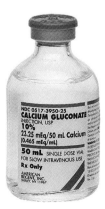
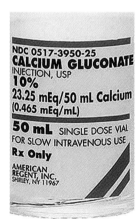

92. CALCIUM GLUCONATE INJ   4.65 mEq

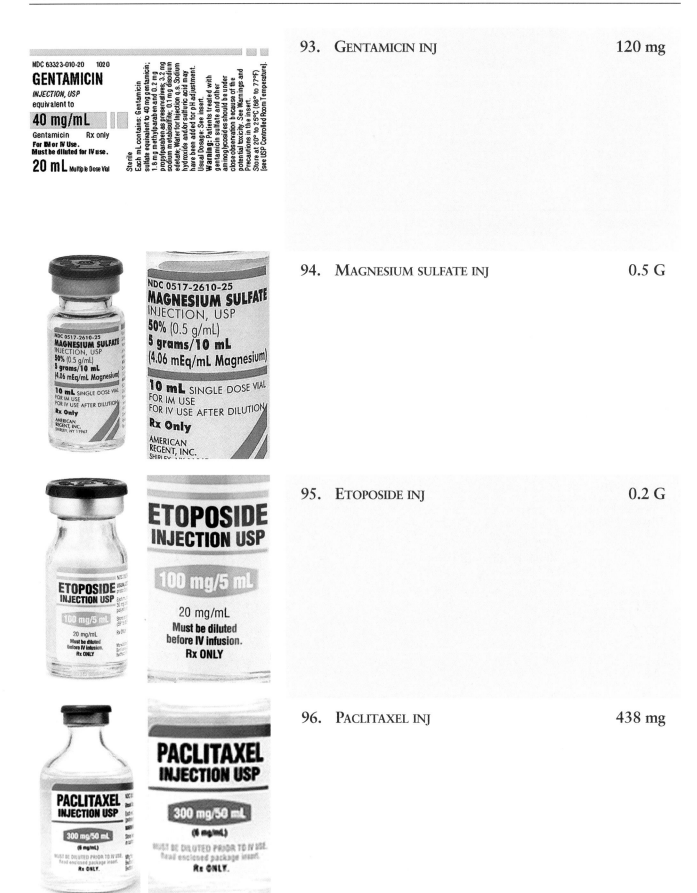

93. GENTAMICIN INJ   120 mg

94. MAGNESIUM SULFATE INJ   0.5 G

95. ETOPOSIDE INJ   0.2 G

96. PACLITAXEL INJ   438 mg

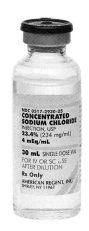

97. SODIUM CHLORIDE INJ   100 mEq

NDC 0517-2930-25
CONCENTRATED SODIUM CHLORIDE
INJECTION, USP
23.4% (234 mg/mL)
4 mEq/mL

30 mL SINGLE DOSE VIAL
FOR IV OR SC USE
AFTER DILUTION

Rx Only
AMERICAN REGENT, INC.
SHIRLEY, NY 11967

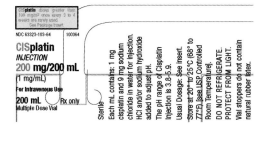

98. GENTAMICIN PED INJ   42 mg

NDC 63323-173-02   17302
GENTAMICIN
INJECTION, USP
(PEDIATRIC)
equivalent to 10 mg/mL Gentamicin
20 mg/2 mL
For IM or IV Use.
Must be diluted for IV use.
2 mL Single Dose Vial
Preservative Free   Rx only

APP Pharmaceuticals, LLC
Schaumburg IL 60173

99. CISPLATIN INJ   75 mg

CISplatin doses greater than 100 mg/m² once every 3 to 4 weeks are rarely used. See Package Insert

NDC 63323-103-64   100364
CISplatin
INJECTION
200 mg/200 mL
(1 mg/mL)
For Intravenous Use
200 mL   Rx only
Multiple Dose Vial

Sterile

Each mL contains: 1 mg cisplatin and 9 mg sodium chloride in water for injection. HCl and/or sodium hydroxide added to adjust pH.
The pH range of Cisplatin Injection is 3.8-5.9.
Usual Dosage: See insert.
Store at 20° to 25°C (68° to 77°F) [see USP Controlled Room Temperature].
DO NOT REFRIGERATE.
PROTECT FROM LIGHT.
Vial stoppers do not contain natural rubber latex.

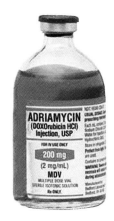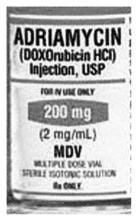

100. ADRIAMYCIN INJ   54 mg

ADRIAMYCIN
(DOXOrubicin HCl)
Injection, USP
FOR IV USE ONLY
200 mg
(2 mg/mL)
MDV
MULTIPLE DOSE VIAL
STERILE ISOTONIC SOLUTION
Rx ONLY

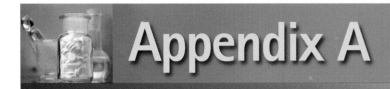
Practice Exam

1. A 10-ml vial of insulin contains 1000 units of insulin. How many ml milliliters are needed for a dose of 20 units?   _____

2. A 500-ml bag of normal saline is set to run at 50 ml/hour. How many minutes will the bag last?   _____

3. A bottle contains 10 g of drug, and the powder volume of the drug is 47 ml. What is the concentration of the drug in milligrams/milliliter when mixed if the final volume is 100 ml?   _____

4. A medication order is written for 500,000 units of penicillin G procaine twice daily administered IM. How many milliliters are required per dose if penicillin G procaine injectable suspension is available in 600,000 units per ml?   _____

5. A 1-L liter bag of normal saline is set to run over 10 hours. What is the rate of infusion in milliliters/hour?   _____

6. A prescription is written for 200 ml of cephalexin suspension 250 mg/5 ml. What is the days supply if the dose is 500 mg four times daily?   _____

7. A prescription is written for a metered-dose inhaler that delivers 200 metered doses. What is the days supply if the dose is two inhalations twice daily?   _____

8. A prescription is written for CellCept 500 mg #100 to be taken 500 mg twice daily. How many tablets can be dispensed within third-party limitations if the third-party plan has a 34-day supply limit?   _____

9. A vial of powdered drug contains 50 mg of the drug. What is the final concentration in milligram/ml milliliter of drug if the powder volume of the drug is 2.5 ml and 7.5 ml of sterile water for injection is added to the vial?   _____

10. Amoxicillin is prescribed at a dose of 50 mg/kg/day in equal doses to be taken every 8 hours. How many milliliters of a 250 mg/5 ml suspension are needed per dose for a 66-pound child?   _____

11. Clotrimazole and betamethasone dipropionate cream contains 1% clotrimazole and 0.05% betamethasone dipropionate. How many milligrams of betamethasone dipropionate are contained in a 30-g tube?   _____

12. Five-percent discounts are offered to senior citizens who get their prescriptions on Tuesdays. What is the amount of the discount for a prescription that would normally sell for $82.24?   _____

13. How many 1-g sodium chloride tablets are needed to prepare 10 L of 0.9% sodium chloride solution?   _____

14. How many 150-mg capsules of clindamycin hydrochloride are needed to prepare 30 ml of a 1% solution?   _____

15. How many 150-ml bottles of amoxicillin 250 mg/5 ml are needed to fill a prescription for amoxicillin 250 mg/5 ml, 2 teaspoonfuls three times a day for 10 days?   _____

16. How many 150-ml bottles of cefaclor 250 mg/5 ml should be reordered if there are three bottles on the shelf and the minimum/maximum inventory level is 4/8?   _____

17. How many 2-ml vials of tobramycin injection 40 mg/ml are needed to obtain 90 mg of tobramycin?   _____

18. How many 500-mg tablets should be dispensed if a prescription is written for metronidazole 500 mg every 6 hours for 14 days?   _____

19. How many grams of 1% hydrocortisone cream should be used to prepare 30 g of 0.5% hydrocortisone cream mixed with Eucerin cream?   _____

20. How many grams of 2.5% hydrocortisone cream should be mixed with 30 g of 1% hydrocortisone cream to make 1.5% hydrocortisone cream?   _____

21. How many mg of certified red color should be used to prepare 0.5 L of a 0.01% solution?   _____

22. How many milligrams of drug are needed for a patient with a body surface area (BSA) of 2.1 m^2 if the dose of the drug is 50 mg/m^2?   _____

23. How many milligrams of drug are contained in 300 ml of a 1:600 solution?   _____

24. How many milligrams of drug are needed to prepare 100 ml of a 1:500 w/v solution?   _____

25. How many milligrams of drug are needed to prepare 300 ml of a 0.1% solution?   _____

26. How many milliliters of 70% isopropyl alcohol should be mixed with 20 milliliters of water to make 50% isopropyl alcohol?   _____

27. How many milliliters of potassium chloride 40 mEq/15 ml are needed for an 8-mEq dose?   _____

28. How many milliliters of 1% lidocaine are needed to deliver 30 mg of lidocaine?   _____

29. How many milliliters of methotrexate 50 mg/2 ml stock are needed to deliver 45 mg of methotrexate?   _____

30. How many valacyclovir hydrochloride 500 mg caplets are needed to prepare 200 milliliters of valacyclovir hydrochloride 50 mg/ml oral liquid?   _____

31. The dose of a drug is 4 mg/kg/day. How many 200-mg tablets should be taken per day if the patient weighs 220 pounds?   _____

32. What is the gross profit (in dollars and cents) for a prescription if the cost of the medication is $38.45 and the selling price is $49.98?   _____

33. What is the percentage strength if 50 ml of a 30% solution is diluted to 300 ml?

_____

34. What is the percentage strength of a 1:25 solution?

_____

35. What is the percentage strength of drug when 80 g of drug are dissolved in 200 ml?

_____

36. What is the powder volume if 80 ml of water are added to reconstitute a liquid antibiotic to make a final volume of 150 ml?

_____

37. What is the rate in drops per minute for a 1 L IV administered over 10 hours if the IV administration set is calibrated to deliver 15 drops per milliliter?

_____

38. What will be the final concentration in milligrams/milliliter of valsartan when eight valsartan 80-mg tablets are crushed and suspended in vehicle so that the final volume is 160 ml?

_____

39. A prescription is written for clarithromycin 15 mg/kg/day for a child weighing 44 pounds. How many milliliters of clarithromycin suspension will be taken each day if an oral suspension containing 250 mg/5 ml is dispensed?

_____

40. For the prescription for clarithromycin in question 39, if two doses are given each day, how many milliliters of clarithromycin suspension will be given for each dose?

_____

Answers to Practice Exam

1. 0.2 ml
2. 600 minutes
3. 100 mg/ml
4. 0.8 ml, – rounded
5. 100 ml/hr
6. 5 days
7. 50 days
8. 68
9. 5 mg/ml
10. 10 ml
11. 15 mg
12. $4.11
13. 90 tablets
14. 2 capsules
15. 2 bottles
16. 5 bottles
17. 2 vials
18. 56 tablets
19. 15 g
20. 15 g

21. 50 mg
22. 105 mg
23. 500 mg
24. 200 mg
25. 300 mg
26. 50 ml
27. 3 ml
28. 3 ml
29. 1.8 ml
30. 20 caplets
31. 2
32. $11.53
33. 5%
34. 4%
35. 40%
36. 70 ml
37. 25 drops/min
38. 4 mg/ml
39. 6 ml
40. 3 ml

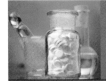

Appendix B

Answers to Practice Problems

1 Numeral Systems Used in Pharmacy

1. 19
2. 90
3. 300
4. 32
5. 44
6. 22
7. 7
8. 4
9. 3
10. 19
11. 33
12. 109
13. 2
14. 8
15. 24
16. 34
17. 43
18. 28
19. 13
20. 29
21. X
22. XX
23. XXX
24. XL
25. L
26. XV
27. C
28. CC
29. CCC
30. M
31. IV
32. VII
33. XII
34. XVI
35. XXII
36. XXXVI
37. XLIX
38. LVII
39. CL
40. CM

2 Fractions: Numerators, Denominators, and Reciprocals

1. 0.5
2. 0.25
3. 0.5
4. 0.4
5. 0.1
6. 0.125
7. 0.083
8. 0.05
9. 0.01
10. 0.001
11. 0.375
12. 0.75
13. 0.8
14. 0.33
15. 0.58
16. 0.143
17. 0.45
18. 0.833
19. 0.22
20. 0.278

21. 0.429
22. 0.273
23. 0.143
24. 0.091
25. 0.143
26. 0.163
27. 0.164
28. 0.206
29. 0.211
30. 0.277
31. 2
32. 4
33. 2
34. 2 1/2
35. 10
36. 8
37. 12
38. 20
39. 100
40. 1,000
41. 8/3 = 2 2/3
42. 4/3 = 1 1/3
43. 5/4 = 1 1/4
44. 3
45. 12/7 = 1 5/7
46. 7
47. 11/5 = 2 1/5
48. 6/5 = 1 1/5
49. 9/2 = 4 1/2
50. 18/5 = 3 3/5
51. 13/3 = 4 1/3
52. 23/3 = 7 2/3
53. 7/5 = 1 2/5
54. 12/5 = 2 2/5

55. 37/5 = 7 2/5
56. 48/7 = 6 6/7
57. 51/7 = 7 2/7
58. 23/9 = 2 5/9
59. 52/11 = 4 8/11
60. 83/23 = 3 14/23

3 Fractions: Reducing Fractions to Lowest Terms

1. 1/3
2. 1/4
3. 1/2
4. 1/8
5. 3/5
6. 1/3
7. 1/3
8. 1/22
9. 1/5
10. 13/15
11. 3/5
12. 4/5
13. 4/3 = 1 1/3
14. 1/5
15. 2/3
16. 3/4
17. 3/10
18. 2/5
19. 4/5
20. 7/18
21. 5/11
22. 0
23. 3/4
24. 2/5
25. 4/5
26. 5/6
27. 1/4
28. 2/3
29. 27/56
30. 2/3
31. 3/4

32. 6/25
33. 1/2
34. 2/3
35. 2/3
36. 12/35
37. 11/14
38. 2/9
39. 3/7
40. 2/17
41. 1/4
42. 1/4
43. 1/6
44. 1/10
45. 1/10
46. 1/9
47. 1/4
48. 1/2
49. 1/3
50. 1/6
51. 1/15
52. 2/9
53. 2/3
54. 2/5
55. 1/2
56. 1/2
57. 1/5
58. 7/15
59. 7/12
60. 3/7

4 Fractions: Adding and Subtracting Fractions

1. 2/3
2. 4/8 = 1/2
3. 1/3
4. 2/8 = 1/4
5. 4/5
6. 4/8 = 1/2
7. 2/15
8. 9/25

9. 5/16
10. 5/8
11. 39/40
12. 4/5
13. 6/7
14. 10/15 = 2/3
15. 10/8 = 1 1/4
16. 11/10 = 1 1/10
17. 31/24 = 1 7/24
18. 35/84 = 5/12
19. 15/12 = 1 1/4
20. 5 703/1000
21. 2/10 = 1/5
22. 1/6
23. 15/25 = 3/5
24. 1/14
25. 4/5
26. 4/20 = 1/5
27. 4/15
28. 343/432
29. 6 31/100
30. 409/1,000
31. 18/10 = 1 4/5
32. 14/8 = 1 3/4
33. 18/12 = 1 1/2
34. 17/18
35. 29/20 = 1 9/20
36. 26/18 = 1 4/9
37. 32/35
38. 41/38 = 1 3/38
39. 47/24 = 1 23/24
40. 23/20 = 1 3/20
41. 20/12 = 1 2/3
42. 17/24
43. 27/24 = 1 1/8
44. 187/198
45. 85/90 = 17/18
46. 10/8 = 1 1/4
47. 12/18 = 2/3
48. 25/36
49. 29/40
50. 15/152

5 Fractions: Multiplying and Dividing Fractions

1. 1/9
2. 3/64
3. 2/9
4. 15/64
5. 3/25
6. 21/64
7. 0/24 = 0
8. 3/20
9. 25/36
10. 8/21
11. 9/16
12. 2/27
13. 1/15
14. 4/125
15. 3/128
16. 7/32
17. 9/40
18. 7/64
19. 4/81
20. 10/1 = 10
21. 7/50
22. 48/455
23. 27/100
24. 0/616 = 0
25. 1/480
26. 3/420 = 1/140
27. 12/1260 = 1/105
28. 3/384 = 1/128
29. 3/168 = 1/56
30. 30/504 = 5/84
31. 6/294 = 1/49
32. 1/480
33. 18/72 = 1/4
34. 15/384 = 5/128
35. 3/378 = 1/126
36. 1
37. 8/24 = 1/3
38. 6/3 = 2
39. 40/24 = 1 2/3
40. 5/15 = 1/3
41. 56/24 = 2 1/3
42. 5/3 = 1 2/3
43. 20/25 = 4/5
44. 16/24 = 2/3
45. 28/8 = 3 1/2
46. 15/24 = 5/8
47. 15/32
48. 4/3 = 1 1/3
49. 144/216 = 2/3
50. 5/75 = 1/15
51. 90/90 = 1
52. 49/25 = 1 24/25
53. Undefined
54. 0
55. 40/72 = 5/9
56. 112/672 = 1/6
57. 56/140 = 2/5
58. 125
59. 300
60. 100
61. 8
62. 25
63. 98
64. 32
65. 49
66. 200
67. 350/3 = 116 2/3
68. 300
69. 800
70. 5,000

6 Decimal Numbers: Writing Fractions in Decimal Form

1. 0.32
2. 0.033
3. 0.237
4. 35.153
5. 503.32
6. 0.86
7. 0.099
8. 0.3
9. 0.014
10. 0.17
11. 6.28
12. 60.028
13. 72.392
14. 850.0036
15. Five tenths
16. Ninety three hundredths
17. Five and six hundredths
18. Thirty two and fifty-eight hundredths
19. Seventy-one and six hundredths
20. Thirty-five and seventy-eight thousandths
21. Seven and three thousandths
22. Eighteen and one hundred two thousandths
23. Fifty and eight thousandths
24. Six hundred seven and six hundred seven thousandths
25. 593 86/100
26. 63/100
27. 75/100
28. 88/100
29. 73/100
30. 2/10
31. 35/100
32. 47/100
33. 66/100
34. 41/100
35. 3/100
36. 1 35/100
37. 3 3/10
38. 4 53/100
39. 6 8/100
40. 10 353/1000
41. 20 354/1000
42. 31 451/1000

43. 49 326/1000
44. 51 118/1000
45. 101 101/1000

 Decimal Numbers: Rounding Decimals and Significant Figures

1. 132.36
2. 6.99
3. 2.36
4. 235,121.35
5. 132,424,324.35
6. 2.34
7. 1.01
8. 3.23
9. 101.23
10. 136.57
11. 80.0
12. 7.6
13. 180.0
14. 37.7
15. 14.3
16. 0.0
17. 3.2
18. 44.4
19. 365.4
20. 0.2
21. 32
22. 56
23. 109
24. 1
25. 100
26. 1
27. 3
28. 3
29. 145
30. 3
31. 4
32. 54
33. 100

34. 325
35. 467
36. 480
37. 513
38. 1,001
39. 2,001
40. 346
41. 4
42. 3
43. 3
44. 2
45. 4

8 Decimal Numbers: Adding and Subtracting Decimals

1. 2.3
2. 11.5
3. 7.55
4. 45.083
5. 72.31
6. 4.6926
7. 276.096
8. 83.315
9. 44.6057
10. 481.25
11. 18.6
12. 25.4
13. 16.5
14. 317.8
15. 956.65555
16. 32.8
17. 1,193.507
18. 36.168
19. 142.3005
20. 245.9853
21. 359.3404
22. 230.4465
23. 5288.5529
24. 22,381.15
25. 56.3404875

26. 1.44
27. 8.93
28. 15.89
29. 0.9757
30. 64.947
31. 4.894
32. 4.7974
33. 30.475
34. 2.9434
35. 34.186
36. 1.68
37. 4.998
38. 1.01
39. 122.999
40. 0.2
41. 145.01
42. 11.1
43. 110.99
44. 109.9
45. 344.02
46. 349.1220
47. 217.5568
48. 5,157.9095
49. 22,369.31
50. 12.1220875

9 Decimal Numbers: Multiplying Decimals

1. 0.42
2. 0.24
3. 0.04
4. 0.09
5. 21.6
6. 38.4
7. 0.42
8. 0.9
9. 0.004
10. 0.009
11. 0.108
12. 0.073
13. 0.0276

14. 0.0225
15. 0.0486
16. 0.0568
17. 0.0006
18. 0.0025
19. 7.4936
20. 223.3
21. 25,899.852
22. 14.52
23. 22.632
24. 7.938402
25. 186.7692
26. 332.212
27. 256.656
28. 5.024
29. 3.66
30. 54.945
31. 512.4
32. 1,784.2176
33. 1,351
34. 14,663
35. 1,235
36. 0.04222
37. 410.161
38. 1
39. 1
40. 779.2876
41. 1064.3808
42. 8.175
43. 1107.1725
44. 2.626745
45. 689.49514
46. 4.03293
47. 0.61
48. 16.06
49. 61.04
50. 155.4
51. 111.1
52. 5.5
53. 2.6
54. 7.5

55. 6.35
56. 5
57. 6.7
58. 66.5
59. 0.9
60. 5.5

10 Ratios and Proportions / Dimensional Analysis

1. a. 5 and 40; b. 8 and 25
2. 6
3. 21
4. 2
5. 14
6. 12
7. 2
8. 1
9. 10
10. 3
11. 2
12. 5
13. 1
14. 6
15. 2
16. 60
17. 1
18. 1,000
19. 8
20. 14
21. 12
22. 20
23. 10
24. 90
25. 180
26. 68
27. 30
28. 20
29. 28
30. 6
31. 15

32. 56
33. 90
34. 102
35. 204
36. 63
37. 136
38. 12
39. 84
40. 21

11 Percents

1. 0.33
2. 0.24
3. 0.333
4. 0.505
5. 0.20
6. 0.47
7. 0.93
8. 0.325
9. 0.75
10. 0.8332
11. 0.6666667
12. 0.185
13. 0.013
14. 0.0025
15. 0.00125
16. 24.44 %
17. 30%
18. 50%
19. 12.5%
20. 75%
21. 2%
22. 9%
23. 10%
24. 80%
25. 36%
26. 52%
27. 40%
28. 65%
29. 2.5%

30. 3.5%
31. 5.5%
32. 0.4%
33. 110%
34. 175%
35. 200%
36. 150
37. 6
38. 3
39. 37.5
40. 3
41. 32
42. 90
43. 1.7
44. 5.5
45. 29.7
46. 2.5
47. 36
48. 20
49. 90
50. 280
51. 80%
52. 20%
53. 87.5%
54. 75%
55. 85.7%
56. 85%
57. 62.5%
58. 42.9%
59. 30%
60. 60%
61. 87.5%
62. 80%
63. 55%
64. 88.9%
65. 50%
66. 10
67. 8.4
68. 4.8
69. 7.5
70. 12
71. 12
72. 50
73. 12.5
74. 27
75. 50

12 Exponents and Scientific Notation

1. 8
2. 1
3. 1
4. 1,000
5. 59,049
6. 46,656
7. 1,728
8. 100,000
9. 256
10. 3,125
11. 9
12. 64
13. 1,296
14. 49
15. 81
16. 100
17. 81
18. 16,384
19. 25
20. 216
21. $1.2 \times 10 \text{ EE } 1$
22. $4.56 \times 10 \text{ EE } 2$
23. $5.309 \times 10 \text{ EE } 3$
24. $7.8322 \times 10 \text{ EE } 4$
25. $1.04043 \times 10 \text{ EE } 5$
26. $1.567334 \times 10 \text{ EE } 6$
27. $1.2 \times 10 \text{ EE } -1$
28. $1.25 \times 10 \text{ EE } -1$
29. $5.6 \times 10 \text{ EE } -3$
30. $8 \times 10 \text{ EE } 0$
31. $1 \times 10 \text{ EE } 2$
32. $1 \times 10 \text{ EE } 3$
33. $5 \times 10 \text{ EE } 0$
34. $1.5 \times 10 \text{ EE } 1$
35. $3 \times 10 \text{ EE } 1$
36. $6.1 \times 10 \text{ EE3}$
37. $7.12 \times 10 \text{ EE } 2$
38. $5.03 \times 10 \text{ EE } 2$
39. $3.5 \times 10 \text{ EE } 1$
40. $1 \times 10 \text{ EE } 6$
41. $0.032 = 3.2 \times \text{ EE } -2$
42. $0.157 = 1.57 \times \text{ EE } -1$
43. $0.0005 = 5 \times \text{ EE } -4$
44. $0.0257 = 2.57 \times \text{ EE } -2$
45. $1 = 1 \times \text{ EE0}$

13 Converting Household and Metric Measurements

1. 1.67
2. 15
3. 946
4. 227
5. 2838
6. 2.5
7. 7.5
8. 11,355
9. 45
10. 59.2
11. 88.8
12. 1,419
13. 1,362
14. 1/5
15. 1.5 or 1.52
16. 3 tsp   1 Tbsp
17. 5
18. 6
19. 2/5
20. 4
21. 2
22. 9
23. 0.22
24. 45
25. 148 or 150
26. 2.27

27. 2.5
28. 946
29. 1
30. 1.98
31. 20
32. 1
33. 2
34. 1
35. 4
36. 8.75
37. 1/2
38. 6
39. 4
40. 3
41. 1.5 or 1½ teaspoons
42. 1 teaspoon
43. 698.86 mg
44. 1/4 teaspoonful
45. 4.56 gal (i.e., 5 gallons must be ordered)

 Converting Apothecary and Metric Measurements

1. 194.4
2. 32.4
3. 1/2
4. 15
5. 2.5
6. 1.852 (rounds to 2)
7. 62
8. 4
9. 6
10. 118.4 (rounds to 120)
11. 16.2
12. 10
13. 88.8
14. 186
15. 129.6
16. 25
17. 59.2
18. 372

19. 1.5
20. 12
21. 2
22. 1/2
23. 3
24. 24
25. 1.5
26. 1.5
27. 388.8
28. 1.25
29. 444
30. 248
31. 1
32. 129.6
33. 40
34. 3,086.4
35. 4.5

 Converting Between the Different Temperature Scales

1. 77 degrees Fahrenheit
2. 59 degrees Fahrenheit
3. 86 degrees Fahrenheit
4. 113 degrees Fahrenheit
5. 50 degrees Fahrenheit
6. 68 degrees Fahrenheit
7. 41 degrees Fahrenheit
8. 86 degrees Fahrenheit
9. 104 degrees Fahrenheit
10. 122 degrees Fahrenheit
11. 72 degrees Fahrenheit
12. 90 degrees Fahrenheit
13. 117 degrees Fahrenheit
14. 36 degrees Fahrenheit
15. 54 degrees Fahrenheit
16. 23 degrees Fahrenheit
17. 14 degrees Fahrenheit
18. 45 degrees Fahrenheit
19. 99 degrees Fahrenheit
20. 64 degrees Fahrenheit
21. 32 degrees Celsius

22. 21 degrees Celsius
23. 0 degrees Celsius
24. − 9 degrees Celsius
25. 27 degrees Celsius
26. 24 degrees Celsius
27. 16 degrees Celsius
28. − 4 degrees Celsius
29. 13 degrees Celsius
30. 38 degrees Celsius
31. − 15 degrees Celsius
32. − 11 degrees Celsius
33. − 6 degrees Celsius
34. 3 degrees Celsius
35. 7 degrees Celsius
36. 14 degrees Celsius
37. 17 degrees Celsius
38. 26 degrees Celsius
39. 28 degrees Celsius
40. 32 degrees Celsius

Calculations for Compounding

1. a. 4 ml   b. 56 ml
2. 15 gm, 1.25%
3. 6 capsules
4. 30 tablets
5. 120 tablets
6. 3 grams
7. 6.2 grams (if 2 oz. apothecary)
8. 25 tablets
9. 12 tablets
10. 10 capsules
11. 2.4 gm
12. 10 ml
13. 10 tablets
14. 7 capsules
15. 30 gm
16. 15 tablets
17. 30 tablets
18. 1 tablet
19. 45 tablets

20. 6 tablets
21. 36 tablets
22. 12 gm
23. 30 tablets
24. 6 tablets
25. 6 tablets
26. 3 tablets
27. 1%
28. 10 capsules
29. 8 ml
30. 0.2 ml

 ## Calculations for Days Supply

1. 30
2. 14
3. 50
4. 10
5. 60
6. 15
7. 100
8. 5
9. 2.5
10. 10
11. 7 (**Hint:** Although the weight of cream in the tube could last for 9 days, the doctor has only prescribed the cream for 7 days.)
12. 37.5–75 days (**Note:** while it is difficult to estimate the exact days supply for this prescription, reasonable answers could range from 15–37.5 days.)
13. 5 (℞ is for 5 days)
14. 15
15. 5 (note, if 500 mg is used per dose, the correct answer is 10 days, if 1 g is used per dose, the correct answer is 5 days)
16. 28
17. 25

18. 2 (**Note:** Assuming the patient would take two tablets, six times per day, the medication would last 1.6 days; however, dosing guidelines for Ultram are not to exceed 8 tables per day.)
19. 30 (**Note:** consider the 16 gm container contains fillers and the 50 microgram amount in the dose refers only to the active drug without fillers.) (**Hint:** To solve this problem, the technician will need to check the package to determine there are 120 sprays per 16 gm container. In this case, the 16 g package size includes fillers. When the doctor writes the directions, the amount of the dose represents only the drug and not the fillers. On p. 82, students are directed to read the package to determine how many metered doses per container. Since there are 120 metered doses per container, the correct answer is 30 days (2 sprays × 2 nostrils − 4 sprays per day).
20. 3 (explanation: for ophthalmic ointments estimate is 100 mg per eye per application is actually 2.2 days)
21. 28
22. 3
23. 60
24. 6 (Prescriptions are written for Medrol Dosepak—take as labeled. To solve the problem, one would need to look up the labeling instructions for the Medrol Dosepak to find the package lasts for 6 days.)
25. 8 (This is a suspension that has approximately 16 drops / 1 ml, so if you use 16 drops/1 ml, the answer is 6 days; however, if you use 20 drops/ml the answer would be 8 days.)
26. 6
27. 25 (**Hint:** Each inhaler contains 100 metered doses)
28. 84
29. 100
30. 10
31. 30
32. 30
33. 25
34. 10
35. 7
36. 15
37. 30
38. 40
39. 30
40. 30
41. 10
42. 30
43. 30
44. 10
45. 10
46. 7
47. 9
48. 10
49. 30

 ## Adjusting Refills for Short-filled Prescriptions

1. 1 box + 8 refills (This is a problem that was added to extend to practical applications in the workplace and only provides the information that is provided by prescribers when they write prescriptions. Nitolingual spray is used to treat acute angina attacks and it is only used occasionally. Because of the nature of the medication, third party

plans would cover one box at a time. If one box would be dispense at a time because of insurance restrictions, it would be necessary to adjust the refills to 8).

2. 5 boxes + 5 refills or 6 boxes + 4 refills

3. 1 bottle + 15 refills (U-100 insulin has 100 ml and each bottle is 10 ml. One bottle would last more than 34 days, so only 1 bottle could be dispensed and the refills would be adjusted to 15).

4. 68 + 2 refills of 68 (leaving a partial refill of 36)

5. 1 bottle + 7 refills (Using 20 drops/ml, and with these directions, each bottle would last more than a month. Insurance would limit one bottle per fill and refills would be adjusted to 7).

6. 1 + 7 refills

7. 1 + 1 refill (The doctor only ordered one bottle with one refill . . . there is no need to adjust the prescription because of the insurance coverage).

8. 1 + 1 refill

9. 68 (since MS Contin is a Schedule II controlled substance, and schedule II medications are not refillable, the patient may want to pay cash for the amount that is not covered by the insurance plan)

10. 34 + 6 refills (leaving a partial refill of 2).

11. 34, 4, 30 (The insurance limit is 34 tablets per RX. Instead of 100, you could only dispense 34, with 4 refills of 34 and one partial refill of 30 would remain).

12. 240, 1, 0

13. 68, 3, 28 (The dose is two tablets per day. 68 tablets would provide a 34 day supply. If 68 tablets would be dispensed per RX, there would be 3 refills of 68 and one partial refill of 28 would remain).

14. 136, 1, 128

15. 500 ml, 3, 0

16. 1 pt., 1, 0 (practical)

17. 136, 3, 56

18. 68, 3, 28

19. 68, 3, 28

20. 34, 10, 26

21. 34, 1, 32

22. 34, 0, 16

23. 34, 1, 32

24. 102, 1, 36

25. 68, 1, 64

26. 34, 4, 30

27. 68, 1, 64

28. 68, 3, 28

29. 68, 3, 28

30. 102, 4, 90

19 Calculations for Dispensing Fees, Co-pays, Difference Pricing

1. $5.00

2. $15.66 ($7.00 + ($12.74 − $4.08))

3. $3.35

4. $25.11 ((0.2 * $12.08) + ($34.77 − $12.08))

5. $5.00 (if the generic is dispensed)

6. $18

7. $40

8. $26.00

9. $28

10. $97

11. $31.20

12. $74.70

13. $40.30

14. $40.10

15. $35

16. $54.50

17. $108.70

18. $44.50

19. $37.90

20. $69.90

21. $32.40

22. $117.70

23. $68.30

24. $101.50

25. $53.60

20 Calculations for Billing Compounds
(NOTE: Your answers may vary slightly due to rounding.)

1. $33.22

2. $17.64

3. $24.20

4. $23.52

5. $21.52

6. $24.32

7. $20.32

8. $34.32

9. $36.95

10. $51.14

11. $16.33

12. $21.22

13. $49.20

14. $16.77

15. $23.17

16. $21.70

17. $17.20

18. $27.32

19. $54.02

20. $32.12

21. $35.02

22. $38.62

23. $37.42

24. $34.15

25. $48.12

 ## 21 Cash Register Calculations

1. 4 pennies, 1 nickel, 2 quarters, 3 one dollar bills, 1 ten dollar bill, 1 twenty dollar bill

2. 3 pennies, 3 quarters, 4 one dollar bills, 1 ten dollar bill

3. 3 pennies, 1 dime, 3 quarters, 3 one dollar bills, 1 ten dollar bill

4. 2 quarters, 2 one dollar bills, 1 five dollar bill

5. 3 pennies, 3 quarters, 2 one dollar bills, 1 five dollar bill

6. 3 quarters, 3 one dollar bills, 1 ten dollar bill

7. 2 pennies, 2 dimes, 3 quarters, 3 one dollar bills, 1 five dollar bill, 2 twenty dollar bills

8. 4 pennies, 1 nickel, 2 quarters, 1 five dollar bill, 1 ten dollar bill

9. 2 dimes, 1 ten dollar bill, 4 twenty dollar bills

10. 3 one dollar bills, 1 five dollar bill, 1 ten dollar bill, 1 twenty dollar bill

11. 3 pennies, 1 dime, 3 quarters, 1 one dollar, 1 five dollar bill

12. 1 penny, 1 nickel, 1 dime, 1 quarter, 3 one dollar bills, 1 five dollar bill

13. 3 pennies, 1 dime, 3 quarters, 1 one dollar bill, 1 five dollar bill, 1 ten dollar bill

14. 2 dimes, 1 quarter, 1 one dollar bill, 1 five dollar bill, 1 ten dollar bill

15. 1 one dollar bill, 1 ten dollar bill

16. 3 pennies, 1 nickel, 2 quarters, 1 one dollar bill, 1 five dollar bill, 4 twenty dollar bills

17. 3 pennies, 1 nickel, 1 dime, 1 one dollar bill, 1 five dollar bill, 1 ten dollar bill

18. 1 penny, 1 one dollar bill, 1 ten dollar bill, 1 twenty dollar bill

19. 1 penny, 1 dime, 1 one dollar bill

20. 1 penny, 1 nickel, 2 quarters, 3 one dollar bills, 1 five dollar bill

21. 1 five dollar bill, 1 ten dollar bill

22. 1 nickel

23. 2 quarters, 4 one dollar bills

24. 2 pennies, 4 one dollar bills, 1 five dollar bill

25. 2 quarters, 3 one dollar bills, 1 five dollar bill

26. 2 quarters

27. 3 pennies, 1 dime, 2 quarters, 3 one dollar bills, 1 five dollar bill, 1 ten dollar bill

28. 1 penny, 1 nickel, 1 dime, 2 one dollar bills

29. 3 pennies, 1 nickel, 1 dime, 2 quarters, 1 one dollar bill, 1 five dollar bill, 1 ten dollar bill

30. 1 nickel, 2 quarters, 1 one dollar bill, 1 ten dollar bill, 2 twenty dollar bills

22 Usual and Customary Price

1. $41.25

2. $17.20

3. $11.00 (*Hint:* ($58.40/100)(12) = $7.00 + $4.00 professional fee for less than $20.00 AWP = $11.00)

4. $312.38

5. $23.95 (*Hint:* ($66.50/100)(30) = $19.95 + $4.00 professional fee for less than $20.00 AWP = $23.95)

6. $5.47 (*Hint:* ($52.43/1000)(28) = $1.47 + $4.00 professional fee for less than $20.00 AWP = $5.47)

7. $6.97

8. $19.38 (*Hint:* ($61.51/4) = $15.38 + $4.00 professional fee for less than $20.00 AWP = $19.38)

9. $7.05

10. $78.91

11. $23.86

12. $33.14

13. $8.44

14. $5.56

15. $4.66

16. $8.32

17. $5.44

18. $5.62

19. $46.98

20. $5.68

21. $11.84

22. $16.10 (for 100)

23. $35.04

24. $270.05

25. $20.86

26. $4.78

27. $16.88

28. $7.73

29. $7.47

30. $11.30

31. $5.64

32. $6.48

33. $7.23

34. $7.13

35. $9.97

36. $7.57

37. $9.31

23 Discounts

1. $4.74
2. $11.85
3. $33.44
4. $85.41
5. $114.45
6. $31.45
7. $86.07
8. $166.35
9. $69.08
10. $213.66
11. $28.98
12. $112.77
13. $242.82
14. $154.38
15. $179.50
16. $355.96
17. $234.85
18. $222.95
19. $294.17
20. $469.20
21. $4.49
22. $11.22
23. $31.68
24. $80.91
25. $108.42
26. $29.79
27. $81.54
28. $157.59
29. $65.45
30. $202.41
31. $303.41
32. $128.51
33. $317.52
34. $213.03
35. $80.06
36. $134.12
37. $210.51
38. $48.78
39. $254.87
40. $108.03

24 Gross Profit and Net Profit

1. $24.46, $18.46
2. $17.18, $11.18
3. $19.90, $13.90
4. $29.31, $23.31
5. $23.63, $17.63
6. $31.39, $25.39
7. $54.06, $48.06
8. $6.71, $0.71
9. $25.59, $19.59
10. $22.63, $16.63
11. $10.19, $6.19
12. $11.19, $7.19
13. $10.19, $5.19
14. $9.19, $5.19
15. $7.79, $3.79
16. $6.00, $1.00
17. $13.09, $9.09
18. $10.19, $6.19
19. $11.19, $6.19
20. $20.79, $15.79
21. $6.79, $2.79
22. $7.19, $3.19
23. $7.19, $3.19
24. $10.19, $6.19
25. $10.19, $6.19
26. $8.14, $4.14
27. $13.19, $8.19
28. $5.79, $1.79
29. $12.19, $7.19
30. $13.19, $9.19

25 Inventory Control

(NOTE: Answers 19–28—The correct answer is 0. None should be reordered at this time because the quantity on the shelf exceeds the minimum inventory level. More product should be reordered and up to the maximum inventory level when the inventory drops below the minimum inventory level.)

1. 1
2. 8
3. 0
4. 11
5. 0
6. 1
7. 8
8. 3
9. 5
10. 4
11. 7
12. 0
13. 3
14. 4
15. 0
16. 0
17. 0
18. 2
19. 0
20. 0
21. 0
22. 0
23. 0
24. 0
25. 0
26. 0
27. 0
28. 0

Daily Cash Report

1.

	Reg 1	Reg 2	Reg 3	Total
+ Cash + Checks	513.12		300.44	**813.56**
+ Bank Charges	120.00			**120.00**
+ House Charges			52.02	**52.02**
+ Paid Outs		5.12		**5.12**
Total	633.12	5.12	352.46	**990.70**
+ Closing Reading	105060.56	21062.12	208121.12	**334243.80**
− Opening Reading	104350.54	20967.00	207768.62	**333086.16**
= Difference	710.02	95.12	352.50	**1157.64**
− Coupons				
− Discounts	8.90			**8.90**
− Voids	10.00			**10.00**
− Refunds				
− Over-rings	56.65			**56.65**
Total	634.47	95.12	352.50	**1082.09**
+/−	−1.35	−90.00	−0.04	**−91.39**

2.

	Reg 1	Reg 2	Reg 3	Total
+ Cash + Checks	1145.63		4322.12	**5467.75**
+ Bank Charges	366.12		980.35	**1346.47**
+ House Charges				
+ Paid Outs				
Total	1511.75		5302.47	**6814.22**
+ Closing Reading	354632.12		17524.82	**372156.94**
− Opening Reading	353099.50		12222.35	**365321.85**
= Difference	1532.62		5302.47	**6835.09**
− Coupons	18.90			**18.90**
− Discounts				
− Voids				
− Refunds				
− Over-rings				
Total	1513.72		5302.47	**6816.19**
+/−	−1.97		0	**−1.97**

3.

	Reg 1	**Reg 2**	**Reg 3**	**Total**
+ Cash + Checks	2002.26		3601.47	**5603.73**
+ Bank Charges	89.12		12.99	**102.11**
+ House Charges				
+ Paid Outs				
Total	2091.38		3614.46	**5705.84**
+ Closing Reading	455325.10		29159.83	**484484.93**
− Opening Reading	453233.55		25543.27	**478776.82**
= Difference	2091.55		3616.56	**5708.11**
− Coupons				
− Discounts			1.10	**1.10**
− Voids				
− Refunds				
− Over-rings				
Total	2091.55		3615.46	**5707.01**
+/−	−0.17		−1.00	**−1.17**

4.

	Reg 1	Reg 2	Reg 3	Total
+ Cash + Checks	1513.12	45.12	2002.02	3560.26
+ Bank Charges	120.00		350.44	470.44
+ House Charges				
+ Paid Outs				
Total	**1393.12**	45.12	2352.46	**4030.70**
	1633.12			
+ Closing Reading	105060.56	21012.12	210121.12	336193.80
− Opening Reading	103350.54	20967.00	207768.62	332086.16
= Difference	1710.02	45.12	2352.50	4107.64
− Coupons	1.10			1.10
− Discounts	8.90			8.90
− Voids	10.00			10.00
− Refunds				
− Over-rings	56.65			56.65
Total	1633.37	45.12	2352.50	4030.99
+/−	**−240.25**	0	**−0.04**	**−0.29**
	−0.25			

27 Parenteral Doses using Ratio and Proportion Calculations

1. 0.15 ml
2. 2.4 ml
3.
   a. 12.5 ml
   b. 1.5 ml
   c. 21 ml
   d. 31.25 ml
   e. 5 ml
   f. 0.5 ml
   g. 4 ml
   h. 0.4 ml
4. 0.5 L
5. 7.5 ml
6. 1 mg
7. 15 mcg
8. 4.7 ml
9. 0.5 ml
10. 1.6 ml
11. 1.75 ml
12. 0.75 ml
13. 0.65 ml
14. 4 ml
15. 15 ml
16. 12.5 ml
17. 14 ml
18. 2 ml
19. 2 ml
20. 5 ml
21. 9 ml
22. 5 ml
23. 4 ml
24. 1 ml
25. 540 mg
26. 1.6 ml

27. 0.5 ml
28. 1.8 ml
29. 3 ml
30. 2.5 ml
31. 8.25 ml
32. 0.6 ml
33. 60 mg
34. 0.78 ml
35. 0.53 ml
36. 2 ml
37. 3.5 ml
38. 0.54 ml
39. 16 ml
40. 0.8 ml
41. 2.16 ml
42. 0.75 ml
43. 36 ml
44. 0.27 ml
45. 32 ml

28 Powdered Drug Preparations

1. 5 ml
2. 45 ml
3. 0.8 ml
4. 8 ml
5. 0.2 ml
6. 500,000 units/ml
7. 92.6 mg/ml
8. 83.3 mg/ml
9. 1.6 ml
10. 11 ml
11. 95.2 mg/ml
12. 200 mg/ml
13. 115.4 mg/ml
14. 4 ml
15. 46 ml
16. 4.6 ml
17. 10.6 ml
18. 130 mg/ml
19. 429 mg/ml

20. 18.4 ml
21. a. 14.5 ml
    b. 2.6 ml
22. a. 0.2 ml
    b. 2.1 G
23. 400 mg/ml
24. a. 3.6 ml
    b. 0.52 ml
25. 19.6 mg/ml
26. 16.8 ml
27. 250,000 units/ml
28. a. 0.6 ml
    b. 0.8 ml
29. a. 0.8 ml
    b. 0.5 ml
30. 1.25 mg/ml
31. A 1 mg/ml; B 10 mg/ml
32. 10.4 ml
33. a. 19.1 ml
    b. 2.4 ml
34. 28.7 ml
35. 1 G/ml
36. a. 1 mg/ml
    b. 0.25 ml
37. Ampicillin 250 mg/ml
    Sulbactam 125 mg/ml
38. 37.6 ml
39. a. 8 ml
    b. 16 ml
40. 2 G/ml
41. a. 0.2 ml
    b. 1.5 ml
42. 200 mcg/ml
43. 1.5 G
44. a. 500,000 units/ml
       (0.5 mu/ml)
    b. 400,000 units/ml
       (0.4 mu/ml)
    c. 250,000 units/ml
       (0.25 mu/ml)
    d. 200,000 units/ml
       (0.2 mu/ml)

29 Percentages

1. 42.5 G
2. 12 %
3. 40 %
4. 75 mg
5. 17 %
6. 2.7 %
7. 14 ml
8. 24 mg
9. 25 %
10. 150 G
11. 100 G
12. 12.5 G
13. 500 mg
14. 3.75 ml
15. 1.25 G
16. 1500 mg
17. 4 caps
18. 4 ml
19. 4 ml
20. 37.5 ml
21. 3 G
22. 80 G
23. 80 G
24. 180 mg
25. 135 G
26. 25 ml
27. 4.8 L
28. 3.75 G
29. 48 G
30. a. 7.02 G
    b. 234 mg/ml
31. 15 ml
32. 908 mg
33. 3 mg
34. 2.5 ml
35. 5.5%
36. 0.4%
37. 8% sulfamethoxazole
    1.6% trimethoprim

38. 4% sulfamethoxazole
    0.8% trimethoprim
39. 15 mg
40. 45%
41. 24 caps
42. 15 tabs
43. 20 ml
44. 1.8 ml

45. 33.3%

 Ratio Solutions

1. 2 G
2. 100 G
3. 125 ml
4. 1.5 G
5. 12.5 ml
6. 1.67 %
7. 375 mg
8. 3.2 ml
9. 0.2 G
10. 50 mg
11. 1:10,000
12. 1:49
13. 0.4 ml
14. lidocaine 200 mg;
    epinephrine 0.2 mg
15. 160 mg
16. 2 mg
17. 0.1 ml
18. 25 mg
19. 20 mcg/ml
20. 1.2 ml
21. 1 mg/ml
22. 10 mcg/ml
23. 0.001%
24. 0.5 ml
25. 75 mg
26. 1:12,500 w/v
27. 2.5 mg

28. 0.05%
29. 1:4000 w/v
30. a. 1:10,000 w/v
    b. 0.01%
31. 187.5 mg
32. 70 L
33. yes
34. 0.02%
35. 0.1 ml
36. 500 mcg
37. 2.2 G
38. 25 ml
39. 2%
40. 75 mg
41. 1:250
42. a. 1:4000 w/v
    b. 2.5 mg
43. 0.0008%
44. a. 5%
    b. 1:20

45. 800 mcg

 Dosage Calculations Based on Body Weight

1. 600 mg
2. 2 tabs
3. 40 mg
4. 6 ml
5. 24.8 ml
6. 981.8 mg
7. 2.5 ml
8. 2 G
9. 1.82 ml
10. 83.3 ml
11. 5.9 ml
12. 3.5 ml
13. 540 mg
14. 0.825 G
15. 10.95 ml

16. 5 ml
17. 242.6 mg; 10 ml
18. 8 mg
19. 9.1 ml
20. 59 mg
21. 2.3 ml
22. 0.3 ml
23. 4.4 ml
24. 4.7 ml
25. 2.8 ml
26. 1.3 ml
27. 0.37 ml
28. 0.96 ml
29. 0.17 ml
30. 3.7 ml
31. 700 mg
32. 106.4 G
33. 370.7 ml
34. 4,128,960 units
35. 2.23 ml
36. 1.39 G
37. 11.8 ml
38. 27.3 ml
39. 43.9 ml
40. 37.2 ml
41. 2.25 ml
42. 70 ml
43. 396 mg
44. 0.6 ml

45. 1 ml

Dosage Calculations Based on Body Surface Area

(Students and teachers should use the nomogram that is in the textbook. To use another nomogram can give different answers.)

1. 72 mg
2. 15 mg
3. 156 mg
4. 11.65 mg